KEEPING HEALTHY IN A POLLUTED WORLD

KEEPING HEALTHY IN A POLLUTED WORLD

HARALD J. TAUB

EXECUTIVE EDITOR, *Prevention*

1817

HARPER & ROW, PUBLISHERS

NEW YORK
EVANSTON
SAN FRANCISCO
LONDON

FIRST EDITION

Designed by Sidney Feinberg

Library of Congress Cataloging in Publication Data

Taub, Harald J
  Keeping healthy in a polluted world.
  Bibliography: p.
  1. Environmentally induced diseases. 2. Environmental health. I. Title.
RB152.T38   1974   614.7   73-14297
ISBN 0-06-014224-3

Contents

vi   *Contents*

Introduction

When a physician reads a book on health by a layman, he is seldom motivated by anything more than curiosity. His assumption, which is for the most part correct, is that he already knows whatever the book has to tell him. If the book accurately reports information familiar to the physician, he considers it is a good job—for a layman.

With regard to this book, however, I feel no inclination whatever to give it a mere professional nod of approval. This book is an excellent volume for anyone, lay or professional, and one from which many physicians have something to learn. The research that Harald J. Taub has put into his work can only be described as massive; and all points toward a new and uniquely helpful approach to the problems of pollution. Awareness of pollution is universal, and we have all read many predictions of coming doom and numerous solutions that never get off the paper. But this is the first work that I have read—perhaps the first one written—that brings the pollution question down to the level of the individual who has to live with it because there is little he is either willing or able to do about it.

It is the only work I know of that effectively presents a wide range of simple, practical measures that any individual can take to protect his health against the onslaughts of the hundreds of inimical materials with which we have contaminated our air, our water and our food.

As a practicing allergist—a clinical ecologist—I am very much aware how subtle and disguised, yet ravaging to health, pollution can be.

Between the clear-cut infectious diseases, which are due to the effects of specific infectious organisms, and those forms of mental diseases related to unbearable mental stress (or deficiencies in body chemistry) there lie an enormous variety of reversible and controllable physical ailments and mental disturbances that result from generally unrecognized allergic, ecologic and addictive disorders. These clinical problems are now diagnosable. Many cases of sinus trouble, headache, arthritis, fatigue, menstrual irregularity, tension, gastrointestinal upset, learning disability, lower-urinary-tract disorder, depression and compulsive overeating and drinking, plus numerous other aches, pains and medical problems, fall into this gray area. When the doctor cannot find a specific cause, he may acknowledge that the difficulty is of unknown etiology. Or he may be one of the large number of physicians who assume that an illness whose organic cause they cannot identify after careful study is probably psychosomatic.

A functional or psychosomatic clinical disorder is one for which there is believed to be no identifiable inciting physical cause or causes. In the absence of a readily discoverable cause, physicians usually conclude that an illness is probably induced by emotional factors, and/or inability to adapt to the realities of our complex modern life. Certainly, no one can deny that some illnesses are caused by psychic or social stresses.

In my personal experience, however, a truly surprising number of ailments stem from exposure to a polluted environment. For example, one of my patients was a twenty-five-year-old woman who showed a variety of symptoms ranging from chronic nasal distress and laryngitis to extremely painful menstruation, fatigue, anxiety and depression. Before she was referred to me, the doctors had thoroughly searched for physical causes and could not actually find any. Although she was first advised to seek psychiatric help, she insisted that the cause of her distress was not emotional but physical. I found out this woman was perfectly right. She was highly susceptible to many of the biologically active chemicals in the environment, notably the hydrocarbons. Many types of commonly used sprays, from disinfectants to hair sprays and air fresheners, could induce or aggravate her symptoms. Fumes from automobiles and buses or trucks, even the gas range in her house, would immediately set off nasal discharge and obstruction; she would experience pressure under the breastbone and feel that there was not enough air in the kitchen, become irritable and feel destructive, sad, tired or withdrawn. The same indoor air pollutants frequently caused nausea, headache, and numbness and tingling of the face, chest and limbs.

In the case of this particular patient, it was fortunately possible to make the necessary changes in her home chemical environment. Faced with the need to get rid of both her gas range and her oil furnace and substitute electricity, she and her family could see the logic of going all the way and moving into a more rural environment, where there would also be less air pollution, including automobile traffic, to contend with. When the indoor and outdoor environmental pollutants were greatly reduced, there was a dramatic improvement in her physical and mental health.

Having treated thousands of such cases, my colleagues in clinical ecology and I are very much aware of how much damage pollution can do and is doing to people even without their realizing it. And while neither Mr. Taub nor anyone else can offer us a universal panacea that will permit anybody to live in a highly polluted environment and emerge from it unscathed, it is probably also true that everybody who takes this book seriously and follows his suggestions will be to some degree healthier because of it.

There are, of course, in the armamentarium of the physician

many medical treatments for the critical ills induced by pollution. These Mr. Taub does not go into, on the sensible premise that if you are suffering from lead or mercury poisoning or have a smog-induced heart attack, you belong under the care of your personal physician. But if the slight dietary additions and changes Mr. Taub's research has uncovered will keep you from ever getting sick with avoidable and preventable forms of illness, physical and mental, you are better off.

I think it quite remarkable that anyone should have been able to compile in a single volume the many ways that scientific research has thus far found by which we, as individuals, can keep some of the worst and most dangerous pollutants from attacking us. When you have read this comprehensive book, I think you will agree with me.

—MARSHALL MANDELL, M.D., D.A.B.P., F.A.C.A., F.S.C.E.
Medical Director, New England Foundation
for Allergic and Environmental Diseases
Norwalk, Connecticut

1   We Love Our Pollution

Pollution and its erosive effects on health are nothing new.

Sketches made 250 years ago by William Hogarth show the bowed legs, bent spines and enlarged heads typical of rickets, the first air-pollution disease.

Directly related to the industrial revolution, rickets was recognized as a common disease in England three hundred years ago, when soft coal was already in widespread use as a fuel. It was the availability of coal that made possible the development of factories and the crowding of laborers into factory towns. The well-known result was the pall of coal smoke that overcast every industrial town and city in England, and Germany as well, with an increasingly dense haze of pollution filtering out the invisible ultraviolet rays of sunlight, and afflicting more children every year with soft bones and the aches and deformities of rickets. Even the animals in the London Zoo suffered from this disease. For two hundred years the treatment of rickets was an utterly unsuccessful and highly lucrative medical specialty.

An article, "Rickets," by W. F. Loomis in *Scientific American* for December, 1970, spells out the history of rickets and pinpoints 1919 as the year by which it had finally become clear that lack of full sunlight was the cause of rickets and that sunlight alone was generally all that was needed to cure the disease. Naturally, the governments of Western Europe, where the disease was particularly severe, took immediate steps to control the release of coal smoke from industrial and residential chimneys and there was a concerted move among city dwellers to relocate in areas where the air was cleaner. Right?

Well, no. In fact, the dwellers in the smoky cities whose children had rickets and whose unborn children were doomed to get rickets, made no effort to remove themselves from the polluted air in which they lived. They went on warming their own homes with soft coal, just as their employers went on running their machines on the heat supplied by coal. And their governments, typically, deplored the problem and did nothing.

What did the medical profession do?

Loomis points out that far earlier the Scandinavians and the people of the Baltic regions had learned that cod-liver oil would both prevent and cure rickets. "By the end of the 19th century," Loomis says, "this therapy had come to the attention of physicians, but it was not generally accepted because a number of variables made the evaluation difficult." In other words, physicians were not going to recommend something as simple as cod-liver oil to prevent rickets until its value was absolutely proven beyond refutation.

Although the nearly perfect efficacy of cod-liver oil was demonstrated in 1917 in a controlled test conducted among Negro children in New York City, a population that, without cod-liver oil, was about 95 percent rachitic, it was not until 1927—ten full years later—that the American Medical Association officially endorsed cod-liver oil for prevention of the bone disease.

I make this point simply to indicate that, even if your doctor does not endorse some of the information in this book, that does not necessarily make it wrong. Much of this material is new, and because experiments on human subjects are no longer considered good medical manners, and experiments on animals indicate only probabilities rather than established truth, it is going to take many years to get some of this material accepted universally. Meanwhile, however, our pollution problems are not going to get much better and may well get worse. Nor are we all going to move to northern Canada, where the air and water remain relatively unpolluted.

In fact, since we're all very human, we may worry about whether the polluted environment is wrecking our health and shortening our lives, and still fight tooth and nail against efforts to remedy the situation. If you doubt that, ask anyone in Seattle how he feels about the banning of the supersonic transport. There is good reason to believe that if there were 500 SSTs flying around the world, the gaseous composition of the stratosphere would be so modified that it would change the character of sunlight and we would all go blind as a result. Dr. Harold Johnson, an authority on atmospheric chemistry, put forward that thesis in *Science* in the issue of August 6, 1971. A panel of the National Research Council, appointed to assess Johnson's arguments, found them "credible," and expressed itself in "general agreement" with his position.

Yet the U.S. government's decision to ban manufacture of SSTs was opposed by the President himself, presumably because of the disastrous economic effect on the Boeing Corporation and, through it, the city of Seattle. Boeing plants have shut down and people have been thrown out of work. Try telling these people that they're better off unemployed than blind. If their comfortable livings and the welfare of their families depend on manufacturing SSTs, they will not and probably cannot believe that there is any valid reason that SSTs should not be manufactured.

Nor have the rest of us any justification for looking down on the unemployed of Seattle. We know, for example, that one of the chief sources of the filth pouring into our air is our own excessive demand for energy. Yet how many of us were willing to sacrifice a little creature comfort to use less energy, until an actual critical shortage of energy left us no choice. The householders of London did not give up heating with soft coal until a new law compelled them to do so. In London it took a killer fog that caused at least 4,000 deaths in 1952 and another in 1962 that killed 750 people in a few days' time to get soft coal outlawed as fuel. When it was illegal, everyone was glad to give it up and persuaded that it was a very good thing to end the sulfurous fogs for which the city had become notorious. Until the enactment of the law, however, there was practically no voluntary abandonment of the cheap but vicious fuel.

The heavy yellow smogs of London, compounded of coal smoke and fog, were obvious pollution that had been going on for at least two hundred years. Nobody did anything about them and few wanted to do anything about them until the situation became crucial. The human race is lethargic about such matters and is likely to stay that way. And if you think that either local governments or the federal government will do anything significant to reduce pollution problems in the United States until a major crisis actually occurs, you're playing roulette against a fixed wheel.

There is, however, one highly noteworthy and often unrecognized point about the London killer fogs. Four thousand people died in one week in 1952, while perhaps another 100,000 were hospitalized for serious respiratory distress and a million more people were unhappily sick at home with coughs, running eyes and noses, and premonitions of doom. That leaves, however, 5,000,-000 people who were little affected or affected not at all.

What made the difference? In 1948 in Donora, Pennsylvania, 5,900 people—almost half the town—became ill during a temperature inversion that trapped the smoke of industrial chimneys. Why didn't the other half?

That is what this book is about.

The first and best thing to do about pollution is either get rid of it or get away from it. But given our own nature and the nature of our social and economic organization, we're as unlikely to do this as we are to ban alcohol or drive the scoundrels out of government. For many types of pollution, however, there are secondary answers—ways to strengthen our resistance and stay healthy—like the vitamin D that is really not quite as good for our health as sunlight, but that will still preserve us from rickets under conditions that keep us from getting enough sunlight.

Do you need such precautions?

If you happen to live on an isolated farm in Nebraska, not too close to Omaha, perhaps not. Most of us, though, live in or near cities, and, whether we realize it or not, are already experiencing a deterioration of health as a result of pollution. If you doubt it—if you happen to think you feel fine—that's just because you're so used to damaged health you don't even know how fine you could and should feel.

Consider your lungs, the abuse they have undoubtedly received, and the effects you already show.

Emphysema may be an unfamiliar term to you, but as a condition you know it all too well. It is loss of stamina because you can no longer exert yourself without becoming breathless. It is sudden spells of coughing that come on for no apparent reason and leave you weak when they stop. It is the bubbly sound of mucus in your windpipe when you talk and often when you merely breathe. Physiologically, it is the loss of elasticity in the walls of the air cells of the lungs. It is brought on by breathing irritating substances.

Once, emphysema was limited to heavy smokers and those who earned their living by working in the midst of pernicious gases or dust—miners, for example. Now it has appeared elsewhere. Everywhere.

In March, 1970, the extent of the problem was described in a speech made by Dr. Russell Sherwin, Hastings professor of pathology at the University of Southern California. Addressing a meeting of the American Society of Clinical Pathologists in Houston, Dr. Sherwin called for strong measures to reverse rising air-pollution levels. If we do not take these steps, he continued, doctors soon might be powerless to deal with various new, obscure lung complaints. Having examined thousands of lungs over the years, he stated that really "clean" lungs no longer exist in people over twelve years of age. "It is not a question whether a person has emphysema," Dr. Sherwin said. "It just becomes a question when it becomes clinically significant. I believe everyone over twelve has emphysema. I know I can't find a normal lung in anyone over that age." So the real question is not whether you have emphysema—you do—but whether it is bad enough to require medical treatment. In a later chapter I will try to show you how to improve your condition. If your emphysema is not that bad, you should welcome the information that will protect your lungs against further deterioration.

In April, 1970, the *New York Times* ran an article on the increase in pulmonary disease fatalities:

The fastest growing cause of death among New Yorkers is pulmonary emphysema, a mortality rate that has risen 500 per cent in the last 10 years according to the New York Tuberculosis and Health Association. During the same period, the association says, deaths from bronchitis have increased 200 per cent.

A city medical examiner talking of the health effects of air pollution puts it more pungently: "On the autopsy table, it's unmistakable. The person who spent his life in the Adirondacks has nice pink lungs. The city dweller's are coal black."

Now take a deep breath—if you dare!—and consider some other figures. In May, 1967, the National Tuberculosis and Health Association *Bulletin* reported that the number of deaths attributed to emphysema and bronchitis doubles every five years. Moreover, it cited surveys made in different areas of the United States showing that at least 3 percent of all Americans over forty have detectable signs of chronic obstructive lung disease. It doesn't take a slide rule to extrapolate from these findings a frightening figure: no fewer than two million Americans were clinically ill with lung disease in 1967. From other quarters have come surveys indicating that one-quarter of the population over forty have anomalous pulmonary function; in plain English, their lungs do not function properly. Again, some quick arithmetic: this translates as about fourteen million Americans suffering from some degree of chronic obstructive lung disease.

And there's nowhere to hide. The National Tuberculosis and Health Association points out that the death rate from bronchitis and emphysema seems to be doubling every five years in *every one of the fifty states.*

Serious as the attack on our lungs may be, however, air pollution is only one of the forms of environmental pollution that is damaging everyone's health.

Although allergies are nothing new, they are multiplying wildly today. Man has filled the world, and ultimately his body, with a dizzying variety of synthetic substances, none of which belong in the human body, all of which are alien to the human constitution. As a result, it's well-nigh impossible to find someone free from one or another form of allergy. Those that cause anaphylactic reaction and histamine production can at least be readily identified. But many environmental allergies do not reveal themselves so typically and may be taken for other types of illness. When they are, they are called "sensitivities." It makes them no less devastating.

Take a symptom, any symptom, no matter how minor. You may think it's something "natural" that will soon go away. Don't bet on it, though. Chances are just as good that it was caused by a sensitivity—to an omnipresent environmental contaminant, to a drug, to a chemical.

Fever can make you uncomfortably warm and flush your cheeks. So can your response to some modern drug or to fumes you breathe every time you ride a diesel bus. At times you may break into a sweat when you haven't been jogging or scrubbing the kitchen floor. The sweat might signal an infection and fever. More often it is a sensitivity reaction. It may be a reaction to sodium nitrate, perhaps, a substance added to most sausages and all canned meats, or to a locally-produced bread containing too much cadmium.

The thousands of unnatural chemicals that invade our bodies daily can be handled by many people without undue stress. There is good reason to believe that in the long run they are harmful to all of us, but in daily life most of us can do a pretty good job of detoxifying them. We'd better. But if you find yourself showing sensitivity reactions too often, you'd better take dietary measures that will improve your ability to detoxify, for keeping away from the offending substance is often a sheer impossibility.

Over the thousands of years of man's life on earth, he has been besieged by a bewildering and enormous assortment of diseases. During this period, his body has developed various ways of withstanding as well as defeating these bacterial or viral invaders. Today, however, the enemy is not so easily recognizable as in the past. In short, when you become ill today, it may have nothing to do with a germ or a "bug." More likely you become ill because of your body's reaction to the unfriendly environment which surrounds us all.

It is a puzzle that has long interested Dr. W. F. von Oettingen of the National Institutes of Health. In his comprehensive book *Poisoning* (Hoeber, 1952), a definitive work on the subject, Dr. von Oettingen compares disease symptoms with poison symptoms, bracketing those which resemble one another and demonstrating that the effects of some poisons may masquerade as signs of familiar diseases. Some of his findings are striking.

Chest pains accompanied by nebulous or intense discomfort and a sensation of tightness are often symptoms of a possible future heart attack or a major respiratory illness. Yet they can also result from mild intoxication caused by various omnipresent chemical substances—the acrolein in diesel exhaust for instance. The same symptoms have also been connected with parathion, the insecticide often sprayed on such basic foods as grains and fruit; ozone, a widely prevalent gas that has been identified as one of the most hazardous atmospheric pollutants; several ingredients of gasoline; and zinc oxide, which goes into deodorants.

If you've ever read about arteriosclerosis, heart degeneration or kidney disease, you know that high blood pressure (hypertension) is a symptom of those problems. But do you know it can also be brought on by inhaling small amounts of carbon monoxide or fumes from leaded gasoline or polluted air?

Then there's your sex life. Perhaps lowered libido, if you're female, or virility, if you're male, can be attributed to natural causes or psychological factors. But such problems can also stem from hydrocarbons in the air you breathe, from the absorption of too much radiation, and *particularly* from stilbestrol, a female hormone used to fatten up poultry and cattle.

It is no exaggeration to call the headache today's most common illness. It may be connected with such serious maladies as brain tumors, but it also may be related to such lesser problems as eyestrain or noise. More often it derives from trying to live normally in an abnormal environment.

Have you ever felt bands tightening around your forehead after sniffing your garden flowers? Of course not. But you may suffer headache symptoms after you've—unknowingly, perhaps—sniffed too much ozone, carbon monoxide, lead particulates or smoke. You could spend the rest of your days searching for a single scientifically accepted case of headache induced by deep breaths of mountain or sea air and never find one. On the other hand, you needn't go very far to uncover stories in the medical literature about headaches brought on by breathing the air that is available to us.

There is hardly a known disease that is not matched, in symptoms and trauma, by reactions to the toxic substances in our environment and our poison-tainted food and drink.

How, then, have we survived? We're eating and drinking and

breathing toxic materials. Why haven't they wiped us all out? Well, some of us *have* fallen by the wayside. Others of us are nearly on the ropes. Yet most are simply limping along, far below the peak of health and vitality, our energies, our mental faculties sapped by scores of ailments—devastating or just a "drag"—born of our environment.

And then there are those of us who are fighting back. They are the ones who meet the insidious poisons of modern life with the kind of vigorous defense and practical antidotes this book will describe. They are exercising intelligently, eating unadulterated foods, improving their intake of special nutrients that speed poisons out of their systems—all of which arms them for this life-and-death struggle.

It's a remarkable world we live in. Technicians, scientists, business leaders have made it so. Thanks to their special skills and frequent genius our lives are far easier than those of our fathers and grandfathers. Yet they are also more perilous. For we can also thank our benefactors for many of our assorted woes. They've worked brilliantly to give us an easier life, but in creating every kind of progress the public will buy, they have worse than ignored—they have actually exploited—the simple fact that we all, at any age, are children in our inability to resist pleasure because it's not good for us. They and we together have created a world far more hostile to human health than it needs to be. We could improve it and we know we should. But what are we doing? We are trying to go on enjoying our polluted world and hoping to stay alive and healthy in the process. It is not an admirable position or even a logical one. But it is human.

You can lower the odds against you with the information in this book.

2 Protection for Your Lungs

The lungs are the gateway to the body—and there is a tiger at the gates.

It has already been pointed out that to some degree all of us have emphysema. Millions of us have chronic bronchitis. We all tend to develop persistent coughs and to react with alarm when our voices start sounding fat and we hear and feel the rasp of mucus in our bronchial tubes.

Really, though, it is when we stop producing mucus that we should get alarmed. These are no longer the good old days when a wet cough was a sure sign of respiratory infection, and your doctor began worrying about pneumonia. In those ancient times, thirty or forty years ago, a woman without seams running up her legs wasn't wearing stockings, and a man without noticeable mucus production had healthy lungs. The times have changed. Today, unless we're on an ocean cruise or vacationing at a well-isolated mountain spot, we are being assaulted with every breath we take. Not only emphysema and bronchitis threaten us, but lung cancer as well.

Lung cancer? You get that from smoking cigarettes, don't you? Sure you do. But . . .

In September, 1972, a panel of the National Research Council

11

reported the results of a two-year study it had made under contract to the Environmental Protection Agency. After surveying just about all published statistics and epidemiological studies, the panel noted with alarm that lung cancer is twice as common among urban dwellers as it is among rural residents. Cigarette smoking alone could not account for the difference, which is obviously more closely related to factory smoke and concentrations of motor-vehicle exhaust. The National Research Council study established that the lung-cancer rate varies within cities, rising rapidly among populations in direct ratio to their closeness to areas of concentration of factories and traffic.

The panel estimates that the death rate from lung cancer rises 5 percent with each additional microgram of benzo(a)pyrene found in 1,000 cubic meters of air.

Let me try to make that figure graphic.

A microgram equals roughly 1/30,000,000 of an ounce. Add that amount of benzo(a)pyrene to the amount of air contained in a room 66 feet square with a ceiling 8¼ feet high, and over a period of years you will increase by 5 percent the amount of lung cancer occurring in that room. This is how potent benzo(a)pyrene is in stimulating the development of lung cancer. And, since this carcinogen is found in cigarette smoke, it is apparent why there is such a close link between cigarettes and the disease.

Yet not all smokers—not even all heavy smokers—develop cancer of the lung. There are many people who can live their entire lives in sections of heavy industry and heavy traffic *and* smoke heavily, and while there is no doubt that their health suffers, somehow they keep their lungs functioning. Why? How?

There are good indications, growing better every year, that the answer lies in vitamin A.

Startling evidence to this effect was unveiled in Tokyo at the Ninth International Cancer Congress, October, 1966. Dr. Umberto Saffiotti, then a pathologist at the University of Chicago Medical School, reported to the congress that in an experimental study he had secured practically 100 percent successful results in preventing chemically induced lung cancer in laboratory animals with vitamin A. The animals Dr. Saffiotti used were hamsters. They were chosen for the very good reason that these animals never develop lung cancer spontaneously. By using them, therefore, the experimenter eliminated the possibility that any tumors arising in their lungs could develop from any cause but the chemical carcinogen Dr. Saffiotti was using on them.

That carcinogen was benzo(a)pyrene from cigarette smoke.

Dr. Saffiotti took the chemical that is invariably found in smoke of any kind and by well-established techniques encouraged the benzo(a)pyrene to fasten to particles of dust. Thus he created the kind of dust found in smoke-polluted air. Bits of the dust were then put into the windpipes of the animals.

It was found that the fluid in the animals' lungs washed the dust particles, separating out the benzo(a)pyrene and dispersing the chemical throughout the lung tissue. Soon the cells began to grow and divide erratically and tumors began to form.

Now Dr. Saffiotti began to feed large amounts of vitamin A to his animals. He found that in many cases the vitamin actually reversed the cancer he had induced, curing the animals that would otherwise surely have died.

Even more important, he found that when he administered large doses of vitamin A, increasing enormously the amount that the animals were storing in their tissues and had circulating in their blood, it was impossible to cause lung cancer in the laboratory animals.

Checking his work in later experiments, Dr. Saffiotti repeated his trials using benzo(a)pyrene alone, without any dust, to eliminate the possibility that the common dust had stimulated the cancer formation. Fifty-nine hamsters had the benzo(a)pyrene administered and were fed 5,000 international units of vitamin A palmitate twice a week. Fifty-seven other animals received the benzo(a)pyrene alone but none of the vitamin.

Among the fifty-nine animals getting the vitamin, there were no tumors in the respiratory tract. The other group developed forty-two tumors in the bronchial passages. This later, confirmatory work was reported to the Federation of American Societies for Experimental Biology in April, 1967.

After this work was done, Dr. Saffiotti was appointed to an important post at the National Cancer Institute and is now working there, in Bethesda, Maryland. Although there is little doubt he is pursuing his studies of vitamin A as a cancer preventive, no public information about his work has been issued since he moved to Bethesda.

What is important now is to apply the Saffiotti discovery to people. But you can't shut people up in cages, control all conditions of their lives, and apply cancer-causing chemicals to their throats. The alternative is the epidemiological study, not altogether satisfactory but still the best way available to test this kind of preventive technique. In such a study you can determine that in a given population—say a city of 100,000 people like Allentown, Pennsylvania—you would expect so many cases of lung cancer over the next ten, fifteen or twenty years. You get everybody in town to agree to take vitamin A supplements every day, and over a period of years you see what effect, if any, the vitamin has on the statistics.

Meanwhile, particularly with regard to a disease like cancer, you say as little as possible about what is being tried. Any publicity is sure to stir up hopes that may be disappointed, which is considered cruel, although personally I cannot see that it is any kinder to leave people without hope. There is, however, a dangerous possibility in unwarrantedly optimistic publicity about a new therapy whose value is not yet confirmed. People may refuse the drastic existing treatments, like surgical removal of a tumorous section of lung, and pin all their hopes on the far-easier-to-take vitamin A, whose effectiveness for people has not been proved. The result could be the loss of many lives that might have been saved. This is a definite danger, and right here I want to warn readers that I do not know and do not claim that vitamin A has any value as a treatment for people with lung malignancies. If you have lung cancer—or if you contract lung cancer six months from now—there is only one sensible thing to do about it. Find a doctor who is an expert in the treatment of this disease and follow his advice.

On the other hand, if you have reasonably healthy lungs and want to keep them that way despite the carcinogenic benzo(a)-pyrene being thrown into the air you breathe by auto exhausts, factory chimneys, home furnaces and a zillion cigarettes, cigars and pipes a day, there is good reason to suppose vitamin A is going to help keep you healthy. Vitamin A does seem to prevent cancer of the lung in people as well as in hamsters.

A report to this effect by Dr. Max Odens of London, "Vitamin A and Cancer," quietly appeared in the German medical publication *Vitalstoffe* of December, 1967, without any ballyhoo or headlines. Yet, the implications of the report are far-reaching. Dr. Odens based his conclusions on both his own research over a period of fifteen years on the effect of vitamin A on bronchitis and the corroboration of the first Saffiotti report in Tokyo.

Vitamin A is necessary to the maintenance of all surface tissues: the skin, the mucous membrane lining the mouth, the throat, the eyelids and outer coat of the eyes, and the mucous membrane lining the respiratory tract, Dr. Odens points out. It was the fact that vitamin A is involved in the maintenance of the mucous membrane lining the respiratory tract that gave him the idea of running a clinical trial and administering daily doses of vitamin A to patients suffering from chronic bronchitis in addition to the usual treatment. He treated seventeen patients, aged forty-eight to sixty-seven, and followed their health for fifteen years. All seventeen patients showed considerable improvement in spite of the unfavorable English climate, and luckily, Dr. Odens says, all of them are still alive, including the oldest. "Even in the severe winters of 1952–53, when there was continuous dense fog and thousands of elderly people suffering from chronic bronchitis died, my patients continued to respond to treatment and were not unduly affected."

It would be remarkable for a group in this age bracket, even in the best of health, to weather fifteen years of the British or any climate without some of them making the obituary columns, but it is even more remarkable in a group seriously afflicted at the outset with chronic bronchitis, often a precursor to cancer.

Dr. Odens suggests that the results of his investigations are sufficiently impressive to warrant serious consideration for the use of vitamin A in the treatment of bronchial disease and suggests, too, that very much the same biological activity of the vitamin which helped his patients overcome bronchitis was at work in the experiments of Dr. Saffiotti establishing the ability of this vitamin to prevent lung cancer in laboratory animals.

How does vitamin A help you to fight infections? Much of its effectiveness is concerned with the cilia, the microscopic hairlike projections of the cells lining the lung's air passages. The cilia perform the necessary functions of trapping and removing from the lung the inhaled foreign substances, including dirt, irritants and potential carcinogens. Without vitamin A, the cilia dry up and lose their function. Vitamin A owes much of its effectiveness to the fact that it restores the cilia to full functioning.

Vitamin A's effect on the cilia was explained as early as 1936 by Sir Robert McCarrison, M.S., Sc.D., considered the father of nutritional sciences, who said in his book *Nutrition and Health:*

Let me draw your attention to the kind of change that is brought about in epithelium by lack of this vitamin. This membrane is covered by tall epithelial cells, each of which has a fringe of cilia. A function of these cells is to secrete mucus which not only traps bacteria but permits the cilia to perform their movements—this they can do only when the membrane they fringe is moist and the moisture contains calcium. The function of the cilia is, by their rapid movements, in waves, to propel bacteria or foreign particles towards the exterior of the body, whence in normal circumstances, they are ejected. It is estimated that the cilia move at the rate of about 600 times a minute. Now when the food is deficient in vitamin A, the cilia slough off and the cells themselves lose their ability to secrete, thus becoming horny or keratinized, as it is called. Figure yourself what this means; no longer is this trapping, this propelling of harmful particles whether of dust or bacteria or both, possible in the areas so affected.

This is information of the utmost importance to all of us, for we are all exposed to air pollutants. If we must inhale these cancer-causing benzo(a)pyrenes, why not fight them with the protective action of vitamin A? It would be like wearing a bullet-proof vest when going into battle—it would not guarantee your survival but it would certainly increase your chances.

Another researcher, Dr. B. K. S. Dijkstra, a Dutch physician, reported in the *Journal of the National Cancer Institute* (1963) that of 330 patients with bronchogenic carcinoma between fifty and sixty-five years of age, a curiously high number were born in March and to a lesser extent February, following a time of year, in the era before modern preservation techniques, when most pregnant women in the Netherlands were poorly nourished. With no fresh vegetables or fresh forage for dairy cows, the vitamin A content in their bodies was low. Dr. Dijkstra stressed the importance of vitamin A in the development of cells such as those in the lining of the bronchi and suggested that vitamin A deficiency is an important factor in the later development of pulmonary diseases. He reported that, more often than not, lung-cancer patients have first suffered from diseases of the lung—caused by poor resistance—such as pneumonia, tuberculosis or asthma.

Dr. Odens has a different explanation of how vitamin A acts to protect the lungs from bronchitis, lung cancer and other respiratory diseases. He maintains that if lysosomes—minute bodies inside the cells containing protein-splitting enzymes—are damaged and if the enzymes leak to the cell substances, chromosomal material could be damaged and this could lead to malignant changes. In other words, vitamin A helps the lysosomes to withstand the effects of carcinogens so that they do not leak enzymes into and damage the cell substance. It is as if vitamin A provided an armor around the lysosome which the carcinogen cannot penetrate.

All right. You should be persuaded by this time that even if you've never smoked in your life, you are threatened with lung cancer if you breathe. How much vitamin A do you need to defend yourself, and where do you get it?

Two well-known authorities on this vitamin, George Wolf and L. DeLuca, both of the department of nutrition at the Massachusetts Institute of Technology, analyzed the Saffiotti studies recently and pointed out that *excess* vitamin A is required under conditions of carcinogenic attack to maintain the formation of mucus-secreting epithelial cells and inhibit the formation of squamous metaplasia (malignant cells).

For a nonpregnant adult the Food and Drug Administration postulates a normal requirement of 4,000 international units a day. Thus we must start out by assuming that to benefit from the anti-cancer activity of the vitamin, we need more than 4,000 units daily. But how much more?

Unfortunately, that question is very much like asking how much gasoline a car needs to travel a hundred miles. We can't begin to answer the question about the car unless we know whether it's a Volkswagen or a Continental, how old it is, whether it needs a tune-up, what kind of tires it has and a dozen other pertinent questions.

And people are a great deal more varied than cars.

Do you do much night driving? Every time your eyes have to adjust from darkness to oncoming headlights and back again, you use up some vitamin A. A man may need more than a woman because he uses it to produce sperm. Broken bones require some of the vitamin for regrowth. A cold uses more, and so does exposure to the kind of chilly, damp weather that produces colds. Some people are able to convert carotene, the orange-yellow pigment of carrots, butter, squash and sweet potatoes, into a usable form of vitamin A within the body. Others cannot. Some convert it partially.

Yet such substantial differences are only minor compared to inborn metabolic differences that exist among people. Nutritional biochemists such as the eminent Dr. Roger Williams have been emphasizing for many years that among individuals the disparities in rates of utilization and in the requirements for various nutrients are so enormous that any attempt to prescribe by formula how much of any nutrient an "average person" needs is the hollowest of mockeries.

My wife will gain weight on eighteen hundred calories a day. Her cousin, whose weight is about the same, will lose on three thousand. How can it be anything but nonsense to try to prescribe by rote how many calories a person needs per pound of body weight? We can do no better regarding vitamin A. It is my opinion that, within the limits of what you are able to take without getting a toxic reaction, the more of this vitamin you secure daily, the better. It serves a variety of purposes aside from lung-cancer protection. It promotes the health and clarity of the skin. If you have occasion to be x-rayed, the vitamin in your system will help ward off any harmful effects from the Roentgen rays. Dr. Henry Sherman of Columbia University has reported to the National Academy of Sciences that giving animals two, three or four times as much vitamin A as they seemed to require for good health brought about greater vigor and disease resistance and longer lives.

So how do you judge how much to take?

First, you must be aware of what a toxic reaction to this vitamin is. The symptoms are deep pain in the bones (which can lead to loss of bone strength), drying and peeling of the skin, itching all over, loss of hair, headache and nausea. These symptoms indicate that you are getting too much vitamin A for your system. They occur in a few individuals who are taking as little as 50,000 international units daily. Most people can take twice that much without any untoward effects. Individual differences again.

Hypervitaminosis A can be a serious matter. Too much of the vitamin over a protracted period of time can damage the bones and the liver. Fortunately, the minor symptoms already mentioned occur first. If you should get any symptoms that suggest a toxic reaction to vitamin A, simply stop taking it for a few days and see whether the symptoms go away. Nutritional authorities state that is all that is necessary to reverse such toxicity. And of course, when you resume taking the vitamin, you will do it at a lower daily intake that you are sure is safe for you.

It is true then, as physicians often warn, that this vitamin is not without its dangers. They are dangers that are easily avoided, however—which is more than can be said for the cancer-causing products of combustion that are in the air wherever large numbers of people live. Remember, the more of the vitamin you can keep in your system without a bad reaction, the better off you are.

There are many food sources of the provitamin, the carotene that is transformed within our bodies. Eggs, dairy products and any orange or yellow plant food will provide it. Fine. Such sources are not reliable, however, to those of us who lack the converting mechanism or who are subjected to certain types of food pollution that make the conversion impossible. On the whole, you are probably better off taking a daily supplement of preformed vitamin A. The fish-liver oils—cod, halibut or shark—are excellent sources, providing the vitamin all ready to go to work on the epithelial tissues of your lungs.

3   Oxygen Can Kill—but Why Let It?

There was a good long stretch of history when a person—at least one who was not utterly impoverished—could get away from polluted air by going to a better climate. It was damp weather, low-hanging clouds, the "closeness" of low-pressure systems that kept smoke contained in a pall of pollution that could be seen and smelled. You knew when the air was bad, and you could take the family to the mountains for a couple of weeks to get away from it. If you felt it was really damaging your health, you could move to California.

Things have changed.

Today, the better the climate, the more dangerous it can be. Thanks to the automobile, it is precisely a Los Angeles, where clouds and rain are rarities and open sky and sunshine are more than abundant, that poses the greatest threat to the lungs and health of its citizens.

That threat lies in oxygen—or at least a special form of oxygen known as ozone. Ozone is formed by the action of direct sunlight on the nitrous oxides that pour out of the exhaust pipes of automobiles. It is pure oxygen. Its chemical formula is O_3. The ozone molecule is, however, unstable and has the special characteristic of promoting rapid oxidation.

21

If there is any doubt in your mind about what oxidation is and what it can do, think of rust. Rust is oxidized iron. Combining with oxygen turns a tough, durable metal into a crumbling, useless powder.

Now oxidation takes place within the human body. Life could not exist without it. Within the individual cell, glucose—sugar—combines with pure oxygen that has been carried to the cell by the blood; the oxidation—the burning—of glucose produces energy and heat.

The process is an orderly one and couldn't be more essential. Suppose, however, that the oxygen enters into an oxidation reaction before it reaches the cell. Then it is no longer available to make heat and energy. Furthermore, the by-products of early oxidation, when it takes place in the blood, can create serious health hazards.

Which brings us back to ozone, a fast-reacting form of oxygen. How fast? Fast enough to produce spontaneous combustion in materials, like oily rags, that would never be ignited by ordinary oxygen. Traces of it will deteriorate and eventually decompose the rubber in your tires. A little ozone in a cream base will bleach hair. It is equally powerful if we breathe it—and we do, if we are compelled to breathe photochemical smog.

More cars and bigger engines in them have led to a chronically smoggy atmosphere wherever the sun shines frequently on a concentration of people. It has been responsible for an enormous increase in respiratory diseases. In 1964, both the American Medical Association and the U.S. Public Health Service issued statements tying a 1,000 percent increase in deaths from emphysema, with concomitant increases in bronchitis and lung cancer, to smog. Ten years later, the situation is far worse.

What happens in the lungs is only the beginning of the damage, for premature oxidation has effects throughout the body. For instance, it causes the formation of peroxides from the lipids—the fats and oils—in the blood. One research scientist, Dr. A. L. Tappel of the University of California at Davis, believes that the oxidation of lipids is responsible for many of the phenomena of aging. Writing in the *American Journal of Clinical Nutrition* for August, 1970, in an article entitled "Biological Antioxidant Protection Against Lipid Peroxidation Damage," he attributes some aspects of atherosclerosis, the arterial disease that culminates in heart attacks, to peroxidation damage. He also believes it damages the liver. In other words, ozone is, beyond dispute, a highly toxic and dangerous gas that those of us who live in areas of photochemical smog cannot escape.

The danger has been recognized since the early 1960s. And since then concerned scientists have been looking for ways we can protect ourselves. One group in the forefront of the search is the Battelle Memorial Institute. Established in 1925 under provisions of the will of the late Ohio industrialist Gordon Battelle, the institute was set up to perform creative and research work, and to direct the use of science "for the benefit of mankind through the processes of technological innovation." Battelle has eight laboratories in the United States, one in Frankfurt, Germany, and one in Geneva, Switzerland. It has six offices in this country, and nine in eight other countries. (The Institute was responsible for important work in the development of xerography and has perfected a revolutionary method of image making using sonic principles that makes it possible to photograph the brain without using x-ray and produce distinct pictures of a fetus with such details as sex and physical condition.)

In recent years the interests of Battelle scientists, particularly at Battelle Northwest, in Richland, Washington, have centered on the search for ways to clean and improve the environment and help man's struggle to survive the pollution that threatens to engulf him. Two years of experiments in the laboratories of Battelle Northwest have led to the amassing of evidence on an important protective role played by vitamin E, specifically as related to the lungs that are exposed to the ozone and nitrogen dioxide in smog.

The studies reveal that animals whose diets were supplemented with vitamin E lived twice as long as those whose diets were not supplemented with E when all were exposed to these two poisonous by-products of the internal combustion engine.

Dr. Jeffrey N. Roehm, a research scientist who worked for a time as assistant and then took full charge of the project, made possible by a grant from the Air Pollution Control Office, told me the experiments with rats showed "very encouraging results" and expressed the hope studies will be extended to human beings.

Prior to that interview Battelle Northwest had announced in March, 1971, at the annual meeting of the American Chemical Society that it had discovered a valuable and practical preventive of the effects of ozone and nitrogen dioxide (the material that produces ozone in sunlight), notably vitamin E.

Three conclusions emerged from the studies on rats, says Dr. Roehm:

1. Vitamin E is a protection against acute toxicity.

2. Biochemical changes occur faster in the lung than in other organs (the lung has surface area the size of a tennis court and of course is first to be exposed to the atmosphere).

3. Ozone results in more rapid depletion of the body supply of vitamin E.

Although emphysema does not occur in animals, the knowledge already gained from the experiments with rats suggests, says Dr. Roehm, that "vitamin E is beneficial in protecting the lung from obstructive lung diseases such as emphysema and edema caused by smog." He told the American Chemical Society's meeting that "vitamin E works as an antioxidant against effects of ozone and nitrogen dioxide on lung tissues. However, vitamin E–supplemented diets will not cure already-diseased lungs, and it appears it will offer protection only to certain levels of ozone or nitrogen dioxide concentrations. Our experiments are designed to *prevent* obstructive respiratory diseases—in humans this means emphysema and chronic bronchitis."

The studies at Battelle Northwest are among the first—yet perhaps the most exhaustive and definitive to date—to determine whether diet can influence the toxicity of ozone and nitrogen dioxide in the lungs. "We started with vitamin E as the most obvious dietary component as a protective agent—something that would modify the effects," says Dr. Roehm. With the usual caution of the scientist, Dr. Roehm declined to make recommendations of how much vitamin E should be used to supplement diet in smog areas, but he did say, "Humans can go ahead and try it; it probably would help them. We know what we have found in the experiments with rats, and we would like to start working with humans."

Such tests would require cooperation from medical doctors, he continued. "Our research with animals won't really do any good until the physician attending a respiratory patient is at least aware of this type of research—that scientists have looked at all the possibilities and there are some encouraging results.

"And that's not the case yet, there is not a general awareness in the medical community that vitamin E might be useful. I get letters from M.D.s and lay people wanting to know what it's all about. It would seem to me that the physician has to be aware that diet may have something to do with the respiratory condition, and that he might recommend to a patient an adequate vitamin E intake along with the other recommendations he makes, such as moving out of the smog zone.

"It should be a preventive thing—if you think you might be subject to a respiratory disease, take a vitamin E pill every day. A significant part of the population has blood below standard; many do not get enough vitamin E."

Exposed continuously to small concentrations of ozone, animals deficient in vitamin E showed mortalities in six weeks. Changes in fatty acids suggested that the same thing that occurs during normal vitamin-E deficiency was occurring in the lung, but at a much faster rate.

"Organs in a body deficient in vitamin E undergo certain changes in fats (lipids), and our body has shown this occurs in the lung, only much sooner. No one knows for sure what happens to the cell structure when penetrated by these oxidants, but we believe that ozone and nitrogen dioxide oxidize the unsaturated fat in the membranous area within cells. The ozone and nitrogen dioxide react with the unsaturated fat, then in turn react with other cellular components such as proteins, resulting in cellular destruction.

"Oxidation is autocatalytic—the overall reaction is very slow at the start, then after a concentration of free radicals is built up, the reaction becomes very rapid. During the period when the reaction is slow, vitamin E is very effective (it traps free radicals, prevents them from building up by absorbing their energy). After oxidation starts, it becomes a chain reaction, and vitamin E stops the chain reaction."

All of which plunges us into one of the most important controversies in science today.

The quoted material is from a thoroughgoing study made over a period of years by a highly competent team of scientists; it concludes that many people do not get enough vitamin E in their diets. It is not the only study to reach this conclusion. There have been hundreds, at least—perhaps thousands. Yet the Food and Drug Administration, which reflects the prevailing medical opinion, insists that everybody gets enough vitamin E and that any kind of dietary supplementation with this vitamin is unnecessary and irrational.

To understand how there can be such difference of opinion in a scientific matter, it is necessary to understand something about what a vitamin is and what kind of role it plays in the human body. A vitamin is a chemical substance found in food which the human body requires for survival, or at least for reasonable health, but cannot synthesize within itself. To make that a little more intelligible, we must understand that there are literally thousands of biochemical materials that our bodies are continually employing in tens of thousands of functions, all thoroughly essential to life and its perpetuation. There are hormones that regulate our ability to function, to rest, to oxidize our food and produce heat and energy, to rise to an emergency, to reproduce ourselves, and to perform many, many other functions, all of which are essential to our condition as living beings.

Then there are enzymes, miraculous chemical substances that have been identified by the hundreds and that probably exist by the thousands. Enzymes induce chemical reactions with an effectiveness and precision that man has never been able to approach in a laboratory. Without enzymes there would be no conduction of nervous impulses, no thought, no digestion, no movement—in fact, no life. We also must, and do, produce other enzymes whose only role is to stimulate enzymes into being, and still others that destroy enzymes when their work is done. They are not vitamins any more than the hormones are, because we manufacture them in our own bodies.

But if the body were not supplied with nourishing materials from food and drink, this vast, bewildering complexity of chemical reactions would simply stop, a condition known as death. The materials we need in large quantities to keep the mechanism going—the proteins and fats and sugars and starches and water, not to mention chicken soup—are what we call food. Food contains not only these gross nutrients, however, but also microscopic traces of other materials that are equally indispensable in ways that are more limited and definable. These are minerals and vitamins. The distinction is that minerals occur in the earth as chemical elements, whereas vitamins are chemical compounds that are synthesized by living things, whether plants, animals or chemists in laboratories.

For example, there is a vitamin called choline. Thus far the only function of choline that has been isolated is its use as one of the building blocks from which the body manufactures a chemical called acetylcholine and an enzyme, acetylcholinesterase, that destroys or inactivates the first one. It is a very limited function, yet if our bodies could not manufacture those two enzymes, we would not be able to transmit impulses along our nerves to crook a finger or chew our food or, for that matter, keep our hearts beating. And, once having transmitted the impulse, we would be unable to shut it off without acetylcholinesterase. In other words, without an adequate supply of this little-known vitamin of extremely limited function, life could not continue. And that, without the tedium of going into the chemical structures and the particular enzyme and glandular systems that are dependent on them, should be enough to understand about vitamins and why they are essential to life, even though we require them in very small quantities.

Which brings us back to the question of vitamin E and how much of this particular vitamin, or any vitamin for that matter, we need. One of the world's great scientists, Nobel laureate Dr. Albert Szent-Györgyi, examines the question in a recent book, *The Living State*. Arguing for a much greater intake of vitamins than the recommended daily allowances endorsed by the National Academy of Sciences and the Committee on Nutrition of the American Medical Association, Dr. Szent-Györgyi takes issue with the medical profession's basic attitudes toward health. He says, "Good health is the state in which we feel best, work best, and have greatest resistance to disease," in contrast to the dominant medical attitude that if you have no discernible disease you are in good health.

There is probably not a single reader who does not know of someone who went to his doctor for a checkup, was assured that he was in perfectly good health, and had a heart attack within the next month. If you mention this recurring phenomenon to your doctor, he will probably react rather blankly and wonder what your point is. As far as he is concerned, the patient *was* in good health until his heart attack occurred. Because the heart attack simply means that a clot of sediment detached itself from the arterial wall and built up in the bloodstream until it cut off the blood supply to the heart sufficiently to induce the death of some of the heart muscle. Nearly everybody has such clots to some extent, and how can anybody predict just when such an event will happen, or say that you're in bad health before it happens?

That is the prevailing opinion. On the other hand, there are some doctors, whose most articulate spokesman is Dr. Wilfrid Shute, a Canadian cardiologist who in his lifetime has treated more than thirty thousand heart patients with remarkable success, who claim that the heart attack results from a deficiency of vitamin E. Vitamin E, they point out, is fibrinolytic, meaning that in the bloodstream it dissolves fibrin, the material in blood that can collect around a clot of hardened cholesterol and calcium, the typical detritus of arterial walls, and build it up until it blocks off the arterial lumen. If you have enough vitamin E circulating in your blood, says Dr. Shute, the possibility of a coronary occlusion is enormously diminished.

Why, then, don't doctors recommend preventive use of vitamin E to try to diminish the swelling incidence of heart attacks, which, according to Lawrence K. Altman in a well-documented feature in the *New York Times* (December 10, 1972), are responsible for 39 percent of all deaths in the United States? Well, for one thing the medical profession is conservative almost beyond belief. The *New York Times* article was written to celebrate the sixtieth anniversary of the first diagnosis in medical history of a heart attack in a living patient. Before 1912, deaths were reported as due to "heart failure," and autopsies did discover the clot or blockage that caused the heart to fail, but it was not until that year that any doctor determined that a still living patient had suffered an interruption of the blood supply to the heart, with consequent damage to the heart muscle. The *Times* points out that Dr. James B. Herrick, who made this significant medical advance, delayed reporting his findings for an entire year because of "the radical nature of the views I held." And Dr. Paul Dudley White, the prominent cardiologist, is quoted as saying, "For ten years, nobody paid any attention to it, not even his own pupils in Chicago. . . . Dr. Herrick said he never knew why. He thought it was an important discovery but the professors of the day never paid any attention to it until about ten years later."

Today the medical profession is, if anything, more conservative. A doctor is constantly haunted by the possibility of a malpractice suit. If he uses any unorthodox therapy not approved by the authoritative committees of his profession, and if his treatment does not turn out well for the patient, he is likely to be sued and to find a jury awarding his patient half a million dollars or so in damages. It is common for lawyers to encourage malpractice suits, and the doctor's only defense is that he treated the patient just as any other doctor would have.

So, when a doctor does try something new, he has good reason to choose a drug that some pharmaceutical company has already spent half a million dollars to test and that has gone through a cumbrous series of animal experiments leading to approval of the drug's use by the Food and Drug Administration. Neither a pharmaceutical company nor anybody else is going to invest that kind of money in testing a vitamin, which you will remember is a substance occurring naturally in food and which therefore cannot be patented and has only a very limited profit potential.

Thus nobody is spending any fortune to investigate the therapeutic properties of vitamin E, and no one is promoting any epidemiological studies to determine whether substantial amounts of vitamin E in the diet will prevent heart attacks or bronchitis and emphysema in smog areas. Biochemists can run their tests and come to favorable conclusions, but as far as doctors are concerned, it is certainly safer to call a patient healthy until he develops chronic bronchitis and then treat him for it. "If, owing to inadequate food, you contract a cold and die of pneumonia your diagnosis will be pneumonia, not malnutrition, and chances are that your doctor will have treated you only for pneumonia," says Szent-Györgyi.

It is sad to reflect that while scientific research keeps uncovering magnificent possibilities for our use of food elements—not only vitamins but dozens of other elements as well—to bring us to "the state in which we feel best, work best, and have greatest resistance to disease," many doctors remain determinedly ignorant of the entire field of nutrition.

This attitude is nowhere more marked than with regard to vitamin E. To find out what is being discovered about this remarkable health-preserving vitamin, you have to read the scientific journals concerned with biochemistry, such as *Science* and *Chemical and Engineering News*. The medical journals maintain a solid silence.

It was in *Science,* the organ of the American Association for the Advancement of Science, that there appeared in August, 1970, a research report by Bernard Goldstein of the Department of Medicine of New York University Medical Center and Ramon Buckley, Ramon Cardenas and Oscar Balchum of the Departments of Medicine and Biochemistry of the University of Southern California, confirming the Battelle Northwest finding that vitamin E protects against the toxic effects of ozone. This report points out what is well known to all biochemists, that vitamin E is *the* natural lipid antioxidant. It interferes with the normal tendency of unsaturated fats to attract atoms of oxygen, bond with them, and, through oxidation, form peroxides.

These scientists took two groups of rats, one of which had been rendered deficient in vitamin E. They then exposed all the animals to a concentration of 10.4 parts per million of ozone. "The 8 vitamin E–deficient rats died of pulmonary edema after 360 to 410 minutes of exposure (mean, 380 minutes). However, all of the control animals were still alive after 440 minutes of exposure, at which time the experiment was terminated." They then ran the experiment again, with the same results. Then they checked again, slightly varying the conditions, to make absolutely certain that they had found what they thought they had. Their conclusion was that the edema—concentration of fluid in the tissues of the lungs—was caused by the oxidation of unsaturated fats normally found in the lung.

It remained for Dr. Luigi DeLuca of the Massachusetts Institute of Technology to tie it all together neatly at a later symposium on pollution and lung biochemistry at the Battelle Northwest facility in Richland, Washington. The most important unsaturated fat in the lung, DeLuca pointed out, is vitamin A. We have already seen that vitamin A is essential to lung health and that a deficiency of the vitamin causes the mucous cells to dry up and harden. Oxidation of vitamin A, DeLuca pointed out, in effect means destroying the vitamin and inducing a deficiency of vitamin A in the lung. Thus, it was agreed, the importance of vitamin E as a protector against smog and its effects may well lie in its protection of vitamin A and its prevention of the destruction of vitamin A by ozone.

In any case, those of us who live in a smog-heavy area need rich supplies of both vitamins; and since defending against ozone tends to deplete them, the worse the smog the more we need. We can't escape pollution, but the double protective action of vitamins A and E can make our breathing a great deal safer.

It remains only to ask which foods are rich in vitamin E. The answer is, unfortunately, just about none. By generous estimates, the average American diet contains about 12 international units a day of vitamin E—a pathetically small amount. Only wheat germ and corn germ are rich in vitamin E. Corn germ is not available and even wheat germ, an excellent food, is not reliable as a source of vitamin E. The reason should be apparent. Vitamin E is an antioxidant and functions as such to prevent the oil of the wheat germ from being oxidized—in other words, from turning rancid. In doing this the vitamin E gets used up.

Things were different when people made their bread out of freshly milled whole-wheat flour. Today there is rarely any wheat germ to be found in your bread, and if you get a special brand containing it, you have no way of knowing how old it is. In the opinion of Dr. Shute, who considers coronary occlusion a vitamin-E-deficiency disease, the deficiency and the enormous increase in heart disease began with the invention of "improved" milling methods that managed to get rid of all the wheat germ.

Under today's conditions, it seems to me, to get enough vitamin E you have no choice but to take a dietary supplement. How much depends on what you want. The biochemists who have been working with protection against smog consider 100 international units a day adequate. To protect yourself against heart attacks, Dr. Shute recommends a starting intake of 100 international units, and then an increase by 100 units at a time, up to a final stable intake of 600 units a day. Vitamin E is not toxic in any amount. The reason Dr. Shute recommends a gradual buildup is that he believes the vitamin increases the volume of blood pumped by the heart, and in cases of very high blood pressure, the sudden increase can be dangerous. Even if your blood pressure is astronomical, however, he has assured me that 100 units a day will do you no harm. If you have ever gasped and choked your way through a temperature inversion that lasted several days, then you already know better than I can tell you why everybody should be trying to protect himself with a good dose of vitamin E.

4   Vitamins Can't Breathe for You

There is a movement under way that will make it impossible for people to take vitamin supplements in the kind of large doses we have seen to be advisable for protection against pollutants in the air. In part, the movement is based on sheer ignorance; in part, it derives from spokesmen for the food industries, which don't want people to think that their breakfast popsy-wopsies lack adequate nutrition; and in part it may be attributed to professional resentment of amateur competition, an attitude many doctors maintain.

A good example of this kind of resentment was recently seen in San Diego, California. A nonmedical but highly professional midwife, with a record of thirty-five hundred successful home deliveries, was charged with practicing medicine without a license. He offered the defense that to assist a healthy woman perform a normal function, without using any drugs, anesthetics or surgical tools, is in no way practicing medicine. The medical testimony in the court case was such that the judge delivered himself of this masterpiece of doublethink:

"Normalcy in pregnancy and birth have nothing to do with health or physiology but only with the statistics of arithmetic. Since 50 per cent of women are not pregnant or giving birth at any given time, normal pregnancy and birth are therefore abnor-malities."

This degradation of the human intellect was perpetrated deliber-ately to convict a man of practicing medicine without a license when it was perfectly obvious to the entire community that his real crime was a phenomenal record of successful deliveries that was superior to that of any obstetrician in town.

So the next time you read—as you surely will—a statement by some pundit declaring that there is no evidence that vitamin A will protect your lungs, I hope you realize you have been pre-sented with the highlights of a mass of existing evidence, and that the pundit just might have motives not necessarily concerned with your immediate welfare. This is not to deny the utter sincerity and dedication of a great number of doctors. As in any business or profession, however, many of the leaders and spokesmen tend to have a very well-developed sense of self-interest.

Nevertheless, although you can discount much of the criticism directed against large doses of vitamins, the critics make one point that is absolutely legitimate. People devoted to vitamin supple-ments do have a tendency to believe they have found the answer to all their health problems. This is simply not so. If you develop bronchitis and think you can simply step up your vitamin intake and not see your doctor you could be making a very big mistake. You could be making an even worse mistake if you let yourself believe that because you're taking 50,000 units a day of vitamin A you can go ahead and smoke with impunity. The vitamin might well keep you from getting cancer or give you a few extra years before cancer develops, but it should not and cannot be expected to give you complete protection against all the kinds of damage that smoking can do to your lungs. In fact, you should not even assume that a protective vitamin intake will permit you to go on forever breathing polluted air without any damage. Bad air is damaging. It is just our good fortune that our bodies are so well endowed with recuperative powers that, given a reasonable chance, they can withstand a fantastic amount of abuse. If you are beaten up by a mugger, you will recover. If it happens every day for a week, it's going to take you longer to recover. And if you're never free of repeated abuse for at least a brief while, it's going to do you in. Your lungs also need a chance to be free of daily abuse for a while, to cleanse themselves and get some rest, if they are to survive as long as they should.

In fact, extreme as it may sound, clean air compressed in cylinders is actually being marketed today. And, while it is undoubtedly a very funny idea, it would do those of us who can't periodically take a jaunt to Lake Tahoe or the Adirondacks a great deal of good to be able to sleep at night in a room full of bottled pure air. This idea was introduced in September, 1970, at a New York symposium on "Air Pollution versus Healing" by Dr. Albert A. LaVerne, a psychiatrist connected with Bellevue Hospital in New York and also editor of the *Physicians' Drug Manual,* the organ of the International Congress of Pharmacology. Don't be quick to dismiss Dr. LaVerne and his strange idea. He has used pure air therapeutically and is surely the country's leading authority on what can be done for health by the real stuff that our great-grandfathers used to take for granted. He believes the long-term answer to the problems created by foul air is, of course, "to cease contaminating our planet if the human race is to survive." But for now Dr. LaVerne insists we need a temporary solution, "a respite from the current relentless and devastating effects of unhealthy levels of air pollution." The temporary answer is pure air, compounded and stored in gas cylinders and available for use as a refreshing substitute for the filthy stuff we breathe every day. Dr. LaVerne envisions the development of inexpensive pure-air units for installation in hospitals, homes and places of work as the immediate answer to the endangered mental and physical health of people who are engulfed by toxic gases and other industrial poisons.

The companies that supply oxygen and other gases to hospitals do sell pollution-free air now—though at a price that is prohibitive to the average person. The pure air is from a low-pollution area or is made synthetically—19.95 percent oxygen, 80 percent nitrogen, and .05 percent carbon dioxide. At the hospital (or home) the tank of compressed pure air is installed in a small room or cubicle which is sealed to prevent polluted air from seeping in. A one-way exhaust fan and a humidifier, though not essential, are beneficial additions to the setup.

Now this is perhaps a more elaborate arrangement (and certainly more expensive) than Dr. LaVerne envisions for the consumer-designed pure air unit he hopes will be developed and which may well be available by the time this is published. As he sees it, a practical unit should be purchasable at a reasonable price and simply plugged in every night to provide pure air during sleeping hours. He tells us why: A group of one hundred New York City dwellers participated in a controlled study on the effects of breathing pure air during sleep. In his paper "Non-Specific Air Pollution Syndrome," presented at the New York symposium, Dr. LaVerne described how a complex of vague symptoms—physical and mental—were improved in patients who were given no medical treatment other than nightly breathing of pure air. There is considerable published research, Dr. LaVerne pointed out, documenting causal and contributory relationships between air pollution and chronic diseases such as bronchitis, emphysema, asthma, heart disease and cancer. However, he added, there is a conspicuous absence of published research dealing with the subtle and chronic effects air pollution has on so-called normal people. The New York study was designed to throw light on this subject.

The "normal" subjects selected for the experiment were not considered "sick." Ranging in age from six to sixty and equally divided between males and females, none had symptoms acute enough to send them to the doctor or psychiatrist. None were on any kind of medical care.

However, when they were interviewed in connection with Dr. LaVerne's research project, they spontaneously described various symptom complexes. "The most frequently described symptoms were headache, fatigue, irritability, lassitude, insomnia, burning of the eyes, difficulty in concentration, and impaired judgment," Dr. LaVerne stated.

Less frequently described symptoms were frequency of urination, perspiration, sweating, epigastric [abdominal] distress, constipation, diarrhea, low back pain. Occasionally described symptoms were "butterflies" in the stomach, continuous state of anxiety, fine tremors, palpitations, sighing. A significant number described impotence, frigidity, premature ejaculation, and other types of sexual inadequacies. The vast majority complained of their specific symptom complexes as being most intense and incapacitating on hot, humid, high air pollution days.

Dr. LaVerne calls this collection of symptoms the "non-specific air pollution syndrome"—or NAPS. How NAPS responds to pure-air therapy was studied in a controlled experiment in which half of the hundred subjects breathed pure air released from storage tanks during their sleeping hours, and half breathed polluted air— that is, the ordinary air of New York City, compressed into tanks. None of the subjects knew which type of air he was getting.

There was no discernible improvement in those who received polluted air. (These subjects were subsequently put on pure air and thus served as their own controls.) On the other hand, improvement in varying degree was noted in 72 percent of those inhaling pure air during the night (7 percent marked improvement, 30 percent moderate improvement, and 35 percent mild improvement). Subjectively, patients noted absence or amelioration of their symptom complexes the next day. Improvement was also measured by objective psychological tests, performed by investigators who, in this double-blind study, did not know which patient received which type of air.

Dr. LaVerne stresses two main points in his crusade for pure-air units. The first, and by far the most important in overall social consequences, is that pollution "diminishes efficiency in most areas of cerebral brain functioning." Since we are a nation (and indeed a world) engulfed by pollution, it would seem disastrous that we must try to solve the world's problems (including pollution) with impaired judgment and unclear thinking. Dr. LaVerne's second point, of most immediate interest to doctors who have read his material and commented on it, is that the healing process is seriously hindered by treating patients in polluted (that is, ordinary) air.

Much of Dr. LaVerne's material on this subject appeared in a thirty-two-page monograph published in the June–July, 1970, issue of *Behavioral Neuropsychiatry*. Let's look at the healing proposition first, and then go on to the larger social issue.

Dr. LaVerne presents limited but persuasive experimental evidence that patients treated in a pure-air environment do better than those in the normal polluted environment. He reports controlled double-blind studies of psychiatric patients and their response to conventional treatment in the two types of air—with clinical improvement notably greater in the pure-air situation. He also reports on a group of sixty patients with acute infectious disease; those who were treated in a pure-air environment showed a significantly more rapid recovery than a comparable group treated in normal polluted air.

He believes the greatest value of pure-air therapy, however, may well lie in its potential ability to restore the thought processes and nervous systems of people who live in high-pollution areas. In his argument for the case he points to the known effects of prolonged breathing of various toxic gases that are found in polluted air. For example, carbon monoxide in concentrations of fifty to one hundred parts per million, breathed for a period of eight hours, "produces deleterious effects of headache, palpitations, ataxia, staggering, impaired intellectual functioning, and other profound central nervous system effects." Gross toxic levels of pollutants reach thirty to fifty parts per million, he says, in such pollution centers as Los Angeles, New York and Chicago, and, in cases of air inversion, soar to 100 and even 150 parts.

Dr. LaVerne suggests that air pollution's effect on the brain and central nervous system may be the cause of "rebelliousness, drug abuse, violence, hostility, suspicion, immaturity, and other adverse behavioral reactions among our youth . . . worldwide." Similarly, he suggests that pollution may be causally related to "the potentially catastrophic disharmony of suspicion, violence, aggression, and war among men and among nations that is rapidly engulfing the world." These are interesting speculations, and not to be discounted, even while we are aware that there are many other factors in our complex technological society that contribute to the ills the psychiatrist enumerates.

Introducing pure air into the immediate environment, as noted earlier, is Dr. LaVerne's proposal for a temporary respite from an intolerable situation, which will not go away until pollution is completely ended. Which may be never. Meanwhile, as good an idea as bottled pure air may be, there is no telling when it will be available at an affordable price. Until then we may have to stick to the best we can get from nature.

Regularly visiting an environment where the air, if not absolutely pure, is still relatively more pure than that of the overcrowded cities where most of us live, is a matter of prime importance. Headaches, confused thinking, fatigue and the other consequences of protracted living in bad air can only serve us badly. Every day we can give our lungs a rest helps. I suggest as a very practical approach fighting for as much vacation time every year as you can possibly manage to get. Then take it a week at a time, spacing it out around the year, and get out where the air is better.

The hardest part of this prescription is resisting the indisputable attractions of such tourist centers as New Orleans and San Francisco, Washington, D.C., Miami Beach and Los Angeles. But stay away from any crowded place. If it's heavily populated, it's polluted. It may not be exciting, but a vacation where there are as few people as you can possibly find, and as much open space, is what is actually going to help with those headaches, restore your ability to sleep at night and the clarity of your thinking, and generally recharge your batteries for the unceasing battle against a hostile environment.

There is just about no damage done by polluted air that cannot be reversed and at least partially rectified by giving the lungs a chance to breathe good air for a while—with one exception. If you suffer from advanced emphysema, clean air alone can't do you much good because you have lost the ability to fill your lungs with it. It's going to take more than vacations to improve your condition.

Emphysema is a rather new disease, whose name was virtually unknown ten years ago. Yet today, thanks to the condition of our air, the spread of the disease is epidemic. There are no exact figures, but well-informed estimates calculate that some fourteen million Americans are affected by it, their numbers swelling by an additional one hundred seventy thousand victims annually. In fact, the Public Health Service finds it very close behind the number-one disabler, heart disease—and it incapacitates more men than tuberculosis, cerebral strokes and mental illness. It causes 30,000 deaths a year and is a contributory cause in 60,000 more.

Emphysema is not a pretty disease. Awake or asleep, the sufferer fights for breath. He cannot empty his lungs enough to pull in fresh air. His days and nights are punctuated with frequent spasms of coughing. His heart is overloaded in its efforts to pump blood through his injured lungs.

There is no known cure. As the disease takes its inexorable course it will transform people blooming with health into gasping invalids who can barely handle even the basics of everyday existence—walking, for example—without a painful struggle.

Yet there *are* a couple of rays of light in this gloomy picture. A specific regimen of exercises, for one thing. It is by no means a cure, but it does get emphysema-stricken lungs into better shape, helping patients return to more or less normal lives.

Perhaps the easiest way to understand emphysema is via a brief anatomy lesson. We can liken the inside of the chest to a major river system. The river itself is the windpipe. Leading from it, one to the left and one to the right, are two main subsidiary streams, known as the bronchi. Smaller auxiliaries, called bronchioles, branch off from each bronchus. They, in turn, end in clusters of air sacs, called alveoli, that look like little bubbles. These alveoli number in the millions and, if separated and laid end to end, they would take up some eight hundred square feet—roughly the expanse of two boxing rings.

Now normal lungs take in about six hundred quarts of oxygen daily—and expel the same amount of carbon dioxide. This is where the alveoli do their job. At each cluster, only a very thin membrane wall separates incoming air from blood. Two-way "traffic" passes through this "curtain"—oxygen and nitrogen on their way into the bloodstream, carbon dioxide and other unwanted gases out to the alveoli.

Abnormal lungs operate in a vastly different way. If emphysema strikes, those thin walls start to disintegrate, and three things happen. First, numerous burst air sacs mass to form larger sacs where air containing carbon dioxide tends to become trapped. Second, each lung starts to lose its natural resilience. Finally, some of the bronchioles find it harder to do their job. They are supposed to move air up and out of the lungs; instead, they develop partial roadblocks, making it harder to exhale the unwanted gases and keep the lungs clear. Not that *inhalation* is blocked. As it continues, however, with more air entering the lungs, that air becomes somewhat "trapped," causing increased pressure. This, in turn, builds larger air traps, known as bullae, within the lungs.

Thus the emphysema patient ends up unable to expel the stale air filling his lungs. It seems as if he can't catch his breath, although his lungs are almost full—of stale air. He must exhale it, and replace it with oxgyen-bearing fresh air. If he cannot, the oxygen level everywhere in his body will continue to drop, since the alveoli just can't carry on their all-important work.

As emphysema progresses, the bronchial tubes and windpipe lose more and more of their elasticity, becoming increasingly flabby and reaching near-collapse. The emphysema sufferer must *squeeze* the air out of his lungs, as if they were an accordion imbedded in his chest. But this only adds to his difficulty because, if he tries too hard to exhale, he will overstrain the walls of the alveoli. Because of the disease, they have become overinflated and resemble a balloon that has stayed blown up too long—they have lost their elasticity and, when deflated, they wrinkle.

In normal lungs, air is expelled through a kind of resilient recoil in a series of spontaneous acts. Day in and day out, the balloon fills up and empties, automatically. Who even thinks about it? No one—except when it becomes less than spontaneous.

As things now stand, emphysema cannot be cured. The disease causes deterioration of lung tissue, and most scientists believe there probably will never be a way to bring new life to dead tissue. So chances are that emphysema may never be cured. The sufferer must learn to live with the disease.

This does not mean there is nothing a doctor can do. I am at the point of describing the best ways I could find, at this writing, that you can help yourself and keep yourself going if emphysema afflicts you. These ways were found and tested by doctors. By the time you read this, other doctors may well have found additional and possibly better ways to aid your condition. In any case, emphysema advanced enough to be incapacitating requires professional supervision.

What the emphysema victim needs is concrete action. And he can start with exercise—an approach that was examined in 1961 and 1962, when Dr. Harry Bass, now head of the pulmonary division of Boston's Peter Bent Brigham Hospital, was with the University of Alabama Medical Center. At that time an increasing number of emphysema victims were seeking help at the center, and conditions were thus right for Dr. Bass to test his hypothesis. He felt that exercise—under meticulously controlled conditions and strict medical supervision—might reduce the total disability that usually awaited emphysema sufferers.

Dr. Bass's subjects were drilled on treadmills and stationary bicycles in a series of exercises that made progressively greater demands on them. Every day they were asked to work a little harder, and most met their rising "quotas." Results were impressive. Of seven men who had been too ill to work before entering this program, two improved enough to return to their jobs. Yet Dr. Bass was not completely satisfied, since program participants were also given oxygen while they exercised.

On transferring to Peter Bent Brigham, Dr. Bass set up a more controlled experiment, which involved bicycle riding alone. His patients now work out on a stationary machine complete with sophisticated electronic circuitry. But improvement on the bicycle —i.e., greater pedaling ability—leads to improvement in walking. As a matter of course, patients who increase their bicycling activity also start walking more—and each one wears a pedometer that proves it!

Admittedly, the whole question of exercise as therapy for emphysema is still somewhat controversial. But let's see how Dr. Bass's patients fared over the first nine years he ran his studies (as reported in the *Journal of the American Medical Association,* December 23, 1969). Eleven emphysema sufferers were enrolled in each eighteen-week program, which consisted of bicycle exercises that became progressively more difficult and demanding. At the completion of each course, Dr. Bass "objectively measured" participants to determine the therapy's effectiveness.

Before being accepted into the program, every participant underwent a complete medical screening. Each suffered from chronic lung disease and, characteristically, found breathing difficult (dyspnea symptoms) when walking at a natural pace on flat ground or while performing everyday activities like washing or dressing. Further, all very much wanted to lead more normal, active lives. And they soon did. Every participant reported measurable, subjective improvement at the program's close, by which point all had stepped up their daily activities.

According to Dr. Bass, objective measurements confirmed those individual reports. New methods of gauging results revealed that there had, indeed, been improvement in pulmonary function. "My patients all have a decreased pulse rate and use oxygen more efficiently," Dr. Bass explained. Emphysema victims who had been house bound could now go for walks, even take in a movie, he added. Dr. Bass is still not sure what caused these dramatic changes. But, he said, "It is probably a combined heart, lung and total body effect. It may be that by decreasing the pulse rate the heart may do as much work with less effort. This is still speculation."

Be that as it may, Dr. Bass's program has meant a new lease on life for many patients. Several years ago, a fifty-year-old suburban Boston housewife who had suffered from chronic lung disease for two decades could walk no more than a few feet—and that only on one of her better days. To all intents and purposes, she was an invalid who could only cross a narrow room by clenching her fists fiercely, taking as deep a breath as possible, and launching herself with those inflated lungs. Less than a year later, after participating in Dr. Bass's program, this same woman was able to walk down several long hallways during a visit to town and spend an hour talking—comfortably, with no difficulty, and keeping within "safe physical limits." As she put it, "I still had a margin of safety."

When another patient, a laborer, first developed emphysema, he was forced to cut his work week in half. After participating in the program, however, he began working full time again.

It is research like this that has helped emphysema patients escape from the limbo their disease has forced them into. Such research does not offer a "cure," but new methods of making life more comfortable and *livable* for the stricken. You can, of course, exercise on a stationary bicycle in your own home and on your own. Don't try riding a bike in the streets with emphysema. There's too much chance you may suddenly run out of breath. But you can do the same exercise in your own bedroom, and expect just as good results.

In London, where pollution has killed thousands, the physiotherapy department in Brompton Hospital and the Asthma Research Council have developed a few simple techniques and exercises, a boon to those with pulmonary malfunction. Brompton credits Winifred Linton, F.C.S.P., superintendent physiotherapist, with developing in 1934 the basic exercises and techniques now used widely all over the world.

More and more physical-therapy departments in hospitals around the country are introducing courses in breathing retraining, the net result of which is to generate confidence in the afflicted individual and enable him to become more active. Instead of being chained to an oxygen tank, people are able to return to a few once-simple chores, like light housework, walking across the street during a green signal, climbing stairs, doing the rounds of stores to shop.

The first necessity—and not exactly an easy task to master—is absolute relaxation of the neck and shoulder muscles. Then the diaphragmatic breathing starts—forcing air out, clear to the base of the lungs, so fresh air can be brought in. There are specific exercises for strengthening abdominal muscles. Pursed-lip breathing is another must—by forcing the air through nearly-closed lips, the bronchi, bronchioles and windpipe open to let the air out. This is not necessarily done all the time, but only when breathing difficulty is experienced.

You learn to coordinate exertion with expiration (exhaling). You breathe *out* if you stoop to tie your shoe or take a step up the stairs. Activity is encouraged—within limits, of course, and under doctor's instructions. Overdoing is as bad as total inactivity.

Learning how to breathe effectively and with minimum effort pays big dividends to the person whose lung capacity has been reduced and virtually lost through disease. Many have learned to do it, throwing off breathing habits of years and following the simple rules taught by doctors and therapists. The beauty of these exercises is that, even if substantial portions of the lungs have been destroyed, they help life to go on at a reduced pace. Also helpful in the retraining process is group therapy—in many communities patients meet regularly, hear from doctor and therapist, discuss problems and progress, share experiences.

It's not easy at first. This program takes plenty of self-discipline, but it's worth the effort, say those who've been through it.

In the following exercises, Figures 1 and 2 illustrate the simple, basic exercise for strengthening the diaphragm, which is all you have left to control breathing once your lungs have lost their elasticity. Figures 3 and 4 demonstrate simple ways to regain control if you get caught in a breathing emergency.

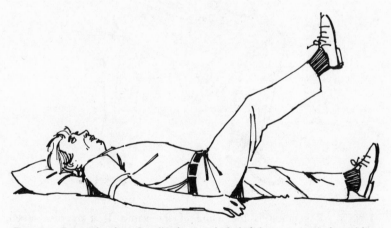

FIG. 1.   Strengthening the diaphragm is helpful to anyone's breathing, but vital to the emphysema sufferer. Raising the legs alternately exercises the proper muscles and aids in expelling air.

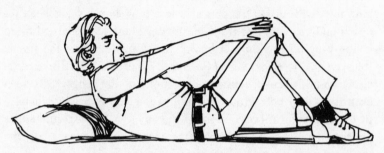

FIG. 2. Bending forward exerts diaphragmatic pressure and helps you to exhale even without lung pressure. Inhale while lying supine.

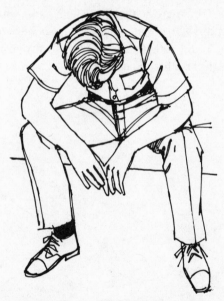

FIG. 3. Relaxation is the name of the game. If a dyspnea attack threatens, sit down, with your hands and head far forward, and breathe out. The position puts pressure on the lungs to expel air. Straightening up will draw in fresh air.

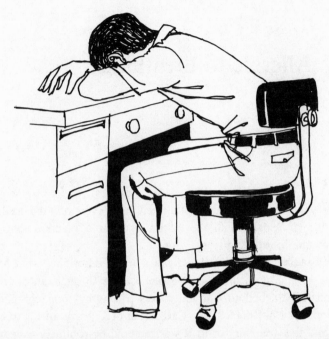

FIG. 4. Another position is shown where patient leans on desk, relaxes shoulders and neck, while doing diaphragmatic breathing. Sitting back again brings about full intake.

It is advisable, of course, to check with a physician before beginning any program of exercises to which you are not accustomed. There could easily be some reason, like a small hernia, why any particular exercise might be dangerous to you as an individual. Besides, he may know even better techniques that have been developed since this was written.

5 Allergic to Breathing

A few years ago, an article published in *Prevention,* the health magazine of which I am the editor, brought a reaction that is truly unique in my experience.

A Canadian woman had sent me a letter describing what she considered her miraculous cure from asthma through nutritional treatment. Attached to her letter was a lengthy mimeographed description by her doctor, Dr. Carl Reich of Calgary, of his treatment and the rationale for it. It was material he routinely gave his patients, I'd guess, to explain why he was treating them in such an unorthodox way. Intrigued, I phoned Dr. Reich, who was reluctant to talk to me but did confirm that he had written the mimeographed presentation I had received and that it was accurate. So I went ahead and wrote an article, pointing out that the treatment had a flimsy basis and was to be considered unconfirmed, although it was still of interest because of its unusual nature. The article was published in September, 1970. During the first week in October, I got a phone call from Dr. Reich.

"What's going on?" he wanted to know. "I've gotten over two hundred dollars from fourteen different people and checks keep coming in nearly every day. They all mention an article in *Prevention.* What the devil have you been saying about me?" I assured Dr. Reich that I had not labeled him a pauper or indicated that he needed any kind of funding. Furthermore, I pointed out, we never brought out an issue that didn't mention at least half a dozen doctors, with descriptions of their work, yet the readers were not in the habit of showering money on them.

When I investigated further, however, it turned out that in this case asthmatic readers were indeed so grateful for the help the information in the article had brought them that a number of them felt they owed Dr. Reich a medical fee and were sending him "payments." As far as I know, this is the only time readers have been so grateful for information that they have insisted on paying for it. And that says a lot about how terrifying an experience an asthma attack is. It is similar to emphysema, with breathing being blocked by accumulations of mucus in the air passages. But an asthma attack comes on suddenly, frequently during sleep, and it can produce sheer panic. Imagine waking up unable to catch your breath, gasping and coughing, and knowing that if you can't somehow clear your respiratory passages in time you can die for lack of air.

Panic at the time and dread of the next attack are perfectly reasonable reactions. If your doctor is willing to leave his bed, he can give you a drug injection (epinephrine) that will quickly end an attack. Since he'd probably rather not—and who can blame him?—he will prescribe drugs for the chronic asthmatic to take when the next attack occurs. They are less effective than injections but they do help, and doctors have to sleep too. If the attack is severe, you may also be rushed to the hospital to be treated by mechanical respirator. Fine. They won't let you die. But, unless your asthma results from one of the well-known and understood allergies like feathers or cat fur, there also isn't much they know how to do to prevent the next attack.

Yet the threat keeps growing, even for those of us who are not chronic asthmatics—and particularly for children. The reason, of course, is that as our air becomes more degraded it contains more and more particulate matter capable of stirring up allergic reactions, even though in many cases the specific allergen cannot be identified. Although there seem to be no statistics available, it is apparent to anyone of mature years that there is far more asthma among children today than there used to be. And a chief reason for it, recent studies have established, is the incredible way the quality of the air we breathe has been permitted to deteriorate. Researchers have known for a long time that filthy air aggravates the condition of asthma sufferers. But new studies are bringing to light some sad facts about the ability of filthy air to *cause* serious allergic disorders in children—so serious that the children affected have to be hospitalized to receive adequate care.

Studies by J. Glaser (*Allergy in Childhood,* Charles C Thomas, 1965) and by H. Arbeiter ("How Prevalent Is Allergy Among United States School Children?" *Clinical Pediatrics,* 1967) show that most allergies in children are already well established by six years of age. And chronic allergic disorders, by far the most common long-term conditions in childhood, are linked, beyond a shadow of a doubt, with one of the most common long-term ailments of our civilization—air pollution. Children may be the most innocent members of our overindustrialized society, but they are its chief sufferers.

One of the first classic studies of air pollution and its allergy-prone victims was made in 1946. It involved American troops and their wives and children stationed in Yokohama, Japan. Researchers found a special form of asthma among the men, wives and children which they called Tokyo-Yokohama, or T-Y, asthma. These asthma cases originated in the heavily industrialized Kanto Plain, between Yokohama and Tokyo, and were clearly correlated with the high level of industrial air pollution in the area. Although the disease did not have all of the usual asthma specifics, patients generally recovered upon moving away from the area.

But most of us can't just move away whenever a factory near our home decides to use our air mindlessly, irresponsibly, as a

garbage can for its wastes. Children, especially, cannot pick up
and go elsewhere (the way troops temporarily stationed in a distant place can) when the filth in the air begins to make them gasp
and heave with asthma. Besides, soon there may be no place left
to go.

"A Study on the Epidemiology of Asthma in Children," (*Journal of Allergy,* St. Louis, June, 1967) by Leonard S. Girsh, M.D.,
Elliot Shubin, B.S., and Charles Dick, M.D., studied the correlation between atmospheric conditions, degree of air pollution and
the number of patients seeking relief from upper respiratory and
asthmatic symptoms. Dr. Girsh and his associates found that elevated barometric pressure and the attendant stagnation of the air
double or triple asthma incidence. And when pollutants and dirt
are trapped in the air—pollutants like oxides of nitrogen, sulfur,
carbon and dust—the asthma rate increases nine times over. These
investigators rather pathetically hope that their study will serve as
a basis for an "asthma index" which will warn clinicians and patients of an approaching peak in the incidence of bronchial asthma.
Now, while an "asthma index" might admittedly be of some help
to asthma sufferers able to flee to a distant mountain peak, it is
certainly not an adequate solution for those who cannot escape
polluted air.

René Dubos, an elder statesman of science, warns us: "Chronic
respiratory disease is now the leading cause of disability . . . in
all the industrialized parts of northern Europe and is becoming
increasingly prevalent in the United States. Air pollution illustrates
how many of the adjustments that facilitate life in a hostile environment commonly express themselves later in disease and human misery."

"An Effect of Continued Exposure to Air Pollution on Incidence of Chronic Childhood Disease" by Dr. Harry A. Sultz and
associates, presented at the November, 1969, meeting of the American Public Health Association, described a study of the incidence
of both asthma *and eczema* in children under sixteen years of

age in the Buffalo, New York, area. All of the cases in the study were severe enough to warrant hospitalization. The results of the study point conclusively to air-pollution levels (measured by suspended particles) as the causative factor. In the nine-year period from 1961 to 1969 the researchers studied 617 hospitalized cases of acute asthma and another 165 hospitalized cases of eczema. Eczema is a terrible, itchy, red skin rash that allergists now refer to as "asthma of the skin." It causes children to lose their appetites and become generally run down.

Here is what the investigators found. In 1969, compared to 1961, there were 86 percent more asthma cases needing hospitalization at the lowest air-pollution level and 114 percent at the highest. With eczema, the average annual incidence of hospitalized cases rose as much as four times in the nine-year period as a result of highly polluted air. Consistently over the nine-year period, an increase in air pollution increased the number of children hospitalized for eczema. The number so hospitalized was 2.9 per 100,000 at the lowest level and 10.2 at the highest. (And remember, these figures represent only those cases serious enough to require hospitalization. What about the untold number of children, never hospitalized, suffering from asthma and eczema?)

E. W. Flensborg has reported a greater incidence of asthma in boys than in girls ("Sex Variations of Cutaneous Reactions in Asthmatic Children," *Acta Paediatrica,* 1956). Other investigators have also shown the greater frequency of boys' sensitivity to scratch tests for inhalants. The Sultz study further confirms the unusually high association between air pollution and the incidence of *both asthma and eczema* in boys. It also points to a much higher incidence of allergic disorders in boys under five years of age than in older boys.

So eczema joins the already long list of diseases linked to air pollution. Childhood allergy and air pollution, in fact, form a vicious circle. Why? Because, though a parent can protect his child from eating foods to which he is allergic, how can he prevent the child from breathing the air? Though he can clean his home of dust and hydrocarbons, how can he clear his house of air? The answer is that short of supplying his child with a miniature gas mask to wear every day (and even that won't really allay the insidious effects of air pollution) he can't. Once the child stops breathing the available air he is, obviously, in serious trouble.

And that is where Dr. Carl Reich and his treatment become of great interest.

Since June, 1967, Dr. Reich says he has treated approximately four thousand cases of the allergic diseases, including bronchial asthma, chronic rhinitis and chronic dermatitis, with vitamin A, vitamin D and bone meal. In over one thousand patients suffering from chronic bronchial asthma, he has successfully resolved the symptoms of 76 percent of his patients, including 90 percent of the children from ages one to ten.

Dr. Reich believes that asthmatic reaction to an allergen involves a nutritional deficiency. In his view vitamins A, D and bone meal work as a team to promote the integrity of the lung muscle and mucous membranes of the respiratory system. If little Johnny wakes up in the middle of the night with an asthmatic attack, the smooth muscle of his lungs is violently contracting, and the mucous membranes of the bronchi secrete an overabundance of mucus.

Vitamin A, you will recall, is one of the cellular components of mucous membrane. Lack of the vitamin will permit, or induce— no one is sure which—the membrane cells to dry up and harden. And most crucial in relation to asthma, the same thing happens to the cilia, the hairlike protuberances on the mucous cells lining the bronchial passages. The importance of the cilia is their motion, similar to that of a stand of wheat rippling in the wind. The motion carries mucus upward in the bronchi, toward the throat. But when the cilia dry up they stop moving, and the mucus stays down.

Doing a little educated hypothesizing, we can describe the sequence. A person breathes in air containing irritating particles of something—say dust—and the lining of the bronchial passages produces mucus, trapping the particles and keeping them from penetrating to the alveoli, where they might get into the bloodstream. Then the cilia move the mucus up to the throat, where you become aware of it and spit it out.

When the cilia become dry and lose their ability to move, however, the mucus stays down and it takes a spasm of coughing to get it up and get rid of it. And sometimes, especially during sleep, a great deal of mucus can accumulate without anything functioning to bring it up to the throat. When it builds up enough to cut off the air supply, the sufferer suddenly wakes up in a panic, gasping for breath and reflexively trying to clear the air passages with convulsive spasms of the lungs. That is an asthma attack, and for reasons we have already discussed, it makes sense for Dr. Reich and others to assert that, for many people, an increased intake of vitamin A should eliminate some attacks and reduce the severity of others.

Reich is far from being the only person to use vitamin A in this way. Dr. Max Odens of London, where bronchial illness is as common as rain, has also published numerous papers about vitamin A treatment for bronchitis. Reich's special contribution is linking the asthma problem to calcium metabolism, and including in his treatment bone meal and vitamin D, both regulators of calcium metabolism.

Unless you are a gardener you may never have heard of bone meal. Widely used as a fertilizer in tulip beds, it is simply the long leg bones of cattle, pulverized. Its special virtue is that, while it is mostly calcium, it also contains phosphorus, magnesium and a number of trace minerals such as strontium, molybdenum and fluoride that are incorporated into bone to strengthen its structure. For human consumption, bone meal is steam sterilized and ground as fine as talcum powder. It is widely available and much safer than the unsterilized fertilizer you feed to your peonies.

To return to Dr. Reich, he has added the bone meal to his

treatment in recognition of the convulsive aspect of asthma. It is
very well known that the circulating blood serum contains a small
but important amount of calcium that is required by all the muscle
tissues, including the heart. If you wake up at night with a cramp
in the calf of your leg, suspect insufficient calcium in your blood.
The same is true of irregularities in the heartbeat, and, in fact, of
all muscle spasms. Calcium lack is not the only cause, but it is a
prominent one.

Why bone meal, then? Why not pure calcium?

That's a good question to which I don't know any hard answer.
Dr. Reich believes that the wide spectrum of additional minerals
in bone meal facilitates the absorption of the calcium. He uses the
vitamin D for the same reason. Many others believe that a calcium lack can be corrected with calcium and vitamin D alone,
without any other minerals, and they may be right.

Whether you try either method, or both, the important thing,
in Reich's opinion, is to keep your bloodstream from going low
in calcium. Then, he believes, you will have less trouble coughing
up an accumulation of mucus and will not get those terrible convulsive spasms of the lung muscle.

Many doctors claim that asthma is psychosomatic. Your son
might threaten to have an attack unless he gets his toy gun, and
scream until he brings on asthma. According to Dr. Reich, this
event represents "the straw that broke the camel's back."

The spectacular effect of emotions is due to the deficiency that
already exists in your son, says Reich. The biochemical alteration
his screaming produces is similar to the alterations of his respiratory apparatus incurred by breathing in irritants with which his
lungs cannot cope. His final anger brought him to the state where
his functions were so greatly altered that he exhibited the signs
and symptoms of asthma. And, by the same token, the removal
of his emotional upsets may result in spectacular remission of his
fits, despite the fact that it played only a minor role.

Further evidence that asthma relates to a deficiency arises when one considers that synthesis of vitamin D occurs in the skin with the help of ultraviolet waves from the sun. Vitamin D is absolutely essential to calcium absorption, which is why a deficiency in that vitamin causes rickets.

Dr. Reich's studies have shown that 75 percent of his adult chronic asthmatic patients had near total protection of skin from sunshine for many years. Furthermore, the asthmatic children almost invariably had been shielded from exposure to the elements during their lifetimes, either by design for reasons of health, or by accident because of the family's way of life. This would suggest that in the relationship between air pollution and asthma the dilution of sunlight might play as big a role as the lung irritants in the air. We do not need a great deal of vitamin D, but we do need some every day. A small daily supplement to make sure of getting enough even on hazy, smoky or cloudy days seems the obvious answer. Too much does carry some dangers, but enough is indispensable.

The chart below lists the quantities of vitamins A and D and bone meal that Dr. Reich prescribes for asthmatic patients. If you do not have asthma but want to take the same nutrients preventively, a third of these amounts should be more than ample.

Daily Intake Averages Dr. Reich Administers

Vitamin D	Vitamin A	Bone Meal
Infant		
1,600– 3,000 I.U.	6,500–22,000 I.U.	¼–½ gm.
Adolescent		
3,600– 5,200 I.U.	20,000–50,000 I.U.	1–3 gm.
Adult		
5,000–14,000 I.U.	28,000–75,000 I.U.	3–4 gm.

Many readers will surely notice that the intake of vitamins D and A recommended here substantially exceeds the amounts suggested by the Food and Drug Administration. The official recommendation, usually accompanied by strong warnings about toxicity, is 400 international units a day of vitamin D, and 4,000 of A.

The discrepancy arises because the FDA is trying, or at least claims to be trying, to protect every last person from the possibility of toxic reaction to the vitamin. There *are* recorded cases of pregnant women who have taken more vitamin D than was good for the fetuses they were carrying—usually prescribed by their doctors, by the way. Since vitamin D promotes calcium absorption, some babies were born with a kidney disorder caused by surplus calcium.

Any kind of toxic adult reaction would be a great deal harder to find. I have pretty good research facilities and haven't been able to find a single case, despite the fact that during the 1930s there were hundreds of thousands of arthritics who took 100,000 to 150,000 units of vitamin D a day, on the advice of their doctors. Sunbathers will easily generate that much of the vitamin in their skins during a day at the beach, and while they sometimes do get severe reactions, they are not to vitamin D.

Thus we have a situation in which pregnant women should be careful to avoid an excess of the vitamin, and should be so warned by their obstetricians. In all probability, new mothers should also be cautioned that when the pediatrician tells them to give the baby four drops of cod-liver oil in his orange juice that doesn't mean a teaspoonful, and certainly not a tablespoonful.

Assuming that the reader is neither a fetus nor an infant, however, there is no reason to suppose any harm can be done by taking five or ten times as much vitamin D every day as the recommended 400 I.U. which will prevent rickets in a normal person. Is there, however, any good reason to take that much?

Well, have you looked at your skin lately?

It has already been pointed out that the growing severity of air pollution is bringing a sharp increase in eczema as well as asthma. Eczema is allergic dermatitis—skin infection arising from external causes such as air containing sulfur dioxide, a pollutant that plays havoc with both nylon stockings and human skin.

As mentioned, eczema has been termed "asthma of the skin," and indeed there is a relationship between the two diseases that is not understood at all, but that certainly exists. Chronic asthmatics have bad skins. Those who suffer chronically from eczema are known to be candidates for asthma. Although it is hard to see why, both seem to stem from the same metabolic abnormality, whether inherited or induced. And both have been equally responsive to Dr. Carl Reich's technique of increasing the calcium intake with bone meal, increasing its absorption with vitamin D and improving its utilization with vitamin A.

So, if you find that your skin breaks out easily and frequently, don't be too quick to blame it on your glands or your nerves. It might just as well be your inability to offer proper resistance to filthy air because you lack one or more of the nutrients Dr. Reich has found we need working together to resist this allergic reaction. And, of the three key elements, the most likely deficiency would be in vitamin D.

Most of us, after all, have learned the advantages of varied diets, with salads and cooked vegetables. We get good amounts of vitamin A in liver, carrots, squash, sweet potatoes, butter and a host of other foods. We get a fair amount of calcium from lettuce, celery, in fact all green vegetables, and more from cheese, and milk if we drink it.

But where do we get vitamin D?

It is becoming increasingly difficult, not to say impossible, to get it from sunlight as the dirt in the air builds up and more thoroughly filters out the ultraviolet rays. And, as a result, vitamin-D deficiency, while no major problem yet, is on the increase.

The only reason that you don't hear much about vitamin-D-deficiency diseases today is that they are rarely recognized by doctors as such, and so, in turn, are rarely reported. Physicians have been taught that there is no longer a vitamin-D deficiency in this country, so they look for other causes. But rickets does exist, and evidence of this was reported in November, 1967, in the *American*

Journal of Clinical Nutrition by Sister Mary Theodora Weick of the Nutrition Department of Mercy Hospital, Buffalo, New York. She found, in studying official records from 1910 through 1961 that 13,807 deaths were caused by rickets, and that from 1956 to 1960, 843 cases of rickets were reported. She doubts that all cases of rickets are reported, and states that rickets "is still noticeably prevalent, and only constant, continual efforts will bring about its complete elimination."

The AMA *Journal* (August 31, 1964) stated that "cases of common nutritional-deficiency disease are being missed because it is assumed they no longer occur and because the diagnostic features have been forgotten. Two examples are outstanding—scurvy (a vitamin C deficiency) and rickets (a disease created by deficiencies in calcium and vitamin D)." The article went on to point out that these diseases are occurring "with disturbing and increasing frequency even under apparently good circumstances and unrelated to other diseases."

When rickets occurs in older people, it is known as osteomalacia. When this vitamin-D-deficiency disease strikes an elderly person, bones that were once hard and straight are bent under the weight of the body and the pressure of muscular activity. Muscles ache and cramp because the distorted position of the bones pulls them out of their normal relationships. In this painful disease, bone structure becomes soft because of an inability of the body to absorb calcium because of a lack of sufficient vitamin D.

A study from England by J. R. Bullamore *et al.* (*Lancet,* September 12, 1970) showed that an aging body often suffers from inefficient calcium absorption, possibly because of a vitamin-D deficiency. Older women, in particular, are susceptible to this condition. The researchers noted a decline in calcium absorption starting at age 55–60 in women and age 65–70 in men. They noted that vitamin-D levels among older women in Britain are low since they receive little of the vitamin from their diet and get little vitamin D from the sun. They add, "It seems reasonable to suppose that for every case of frank osteomalacia there are many cases of subclinical vitamin D deficiency with malabsorption of calcium which are not yet recognized."

The same journal in 1966 published a study by A. N. Exton-Smith, H. M. Hodkinson and B. R. Stanton, who found a strong relationship between low bone density in elderly women and low intakes of vitamin D. They suggested that an unsuspected dietary deficiency of vitamin D may be an important factor in the production of skeletal rarefaction in the elderly.

Part of the problem is that the sources of vitamin D are fewer than those of any other vitamin. There are only three of them— a synthetic one, and two natural sources.

The synthetic source is milk. One must drink a full quart of irradiated whole milk or its equivalent in nonfat dry milk to obtain the minimum requirement of 400 I.U. Nutritionists who have encouraged people to let down their guard by assuring them that rickets is a thing of the past because of the availability of irradiated milk are unfairly ignoring the facts. About half of the population, because of allergic reactions, inability to digest milk, or simply because of taste, do not drink more than a few ounces of milk a day, if they drink it at all!

A majority of adults find milk intolerable. For example, most Negroes and Orientals have a hereditary lack of the enzyme lactase, and without this enzyme are unable to drink milk without digestive discomfort followed by diarrhea. Many Caucasians also, as they grow older, stop producing lactase and become unable to digest milk. Besides, on a wider scale, irradiated milk is not available even to the people of most of the developed nations throughout the world.

Vitamin-D deficiency can occur at any age. According to a study reported in the *Quarterly Journal of Medicine* (38: 195–209, 1969) by C. E. Dent and R. Smith at the University College Hospital Medical School, London, the impression that dietary deficiencies as a cause of rickets or osteomalacia applies only to children or old people is erroneous. These investigators found nutritional osteomalacia in seven adult women between the ages of twenty and forty-six. When you consider the extreme measures that many women take to lose weight, cutting out most nutritional foods, and neglecting to supplement their diets with the necessary vitamins, it becomes apparent that they *can* become vulnerable to osteomalacia. Not only that, but the same study showed that in two of the seven patients the disease recurred eight and ten years later.

The current environmental crisis, which is every day growing worse, probably has a great deal to do with the fact that rickets and osteomalacia are again being recognized. The reason is the very one that was responsible for rickets three hundred years ago— air pollution. Only this time it is on a much wider scale, making the problem much more serious. Once again smoke has filled the skies, only this time there are thousands more smokestacks; once again cities are crowded, but this time there are even more people, and even taller buildings; and worst of all, now there are automobiles, every one of which is spewing its own soot into the air, throwing up a smoke screen against the prime source of vitamin D.

More than fifty years ago people learned that the way to stop vitamin-D-deficiency diseases when sunlight was not available was to make sure that they got enough fish or fish-liver oil. When they did, the disease disappeared. The same technique must be applied again today.

In the face of a growing air-pollution problem the one sure way to avoid vitamin-D-deficiency diseases is to supplement your diet with fish-liver oils. They are natural and safe, and can be taken in seconds in convenient tiny capsules. It's a fast and easy way to get rid of those winter aches in the bones and to stop feeling old. Combined with otherwise good nutrition, it should also improve your chances of keeping a clear skin and clear lungs.

6   Let the Light Shine In

Sunlight, and particularly its ultraviolet spectrum, has a lot more effect on us than simply generating vitamin D. And the dwindling of the number of days in a year when we are able to receive the full spectrum of sunlight may well be affecting health in ways that have nothing to do with how little vitamin D we are getting. Other profound effects of light on the way we function depend simply and directly on how much light passes through our eyes and the wavelengths that make up that light.

The eye as the window of the soul may be no more than a flight of poetic fancy, but it is hard fact that the eye is the window of two ultimately important glands—the pineal and the body's master gland, the pituitary. Both these glands seem to be programmed to function in response to how much or how little light they receive through the eye. There is good reason to believe that even a minor change in the quality of light, such as the filtering of ultraviolet by smog or factory smoke, can induce profound changes in both the quantity of hormones the body produces and when it produces them, all of which in its turn can have profound effects on our bodies and how they function.

How profound?

Consider the experience of John Ott with arthritis, an experience that has completely reoriented the life and work of this highly creative scientist-technician. John Nash Ott, Ph.D., is a man well known in film circles. He is the original developer and pioneer of time-lapse photography, the technique by which the screen can show flowers actually growing. You saw some of his work in *On a Clear Day You Can See Forever,* as well as in a number of Disney nature films. A brilliant technician, he was so badly crippled by arthritis in his hips that he nearly had to stop working. He walked with a cane and was told he would have to wear metal braces if he was ever to stand upright again.

One of the folk remedies for arthritis is sunbathing. Until recently, orthopedic physicians had no glimmer of an idea of why sunbathing should have any effect whatsoever on the arthritic condition, yet they acknowledge that many thousands of arthritis sufferers do feel less pain and have greater mobility when they sunbathe, even though just as many others are not helped at all. Dr. Ott's physician encouraged him to try the sun. He didn't know any other way to help him.

Ott was desperate enough to be willing to give up working and spend his days on a beach, if that would only ease the pain he suffered continually. He left Chicago and moved to Sarasota, Florida, where he could get out in the sunshine the year round. Wearing only sunglasses and trunks he exposed himself day after day on the Sarasota beach—and it didn't help him one bit.

One day the sunglasses were accidentally broken. Ott continued to go out on the beach without them, though the glare troubled his eyes. Within a few days he believed that he noticed a dramatic improvement in his condition. When he was able to throw away his cane, he was certain. The arthritic condition had been improved by sunlight, but not, as is generally thought, by the action of sunlight on the skin. It was by acting on the system through the eyes, he now felt, that the sunlight had vastly benefited his health.

Ott was well equipped to investigate further. First he checked the sunglasses he had worn, to determine which portions of the natural sunlight they had filtered out. The answer, it turned out, was that the glasses had filtered out both the ultraviolet and the long infrared rays of the sunlight. Next was a check on the medical literature. There was little to be found, but there was one research scientist—Dr. Richard Wurtman—who had done a great deal of work in the area. Now professor of endocrinology and metabolism at Massachusetts Institute of Technology, Dr. Wurtman had formerly been at the National Institutes of Health, where he had intensively investigated the effect of light on the pituitary and the pineal glands, finding that both these glands of the brain were stimulated by ultraviolet light entering the eye. Key glands in the entire human endocrine structure, the pituitary and pineal not only play their own roles in control of such basic functions as growth and maturation, but their hormone secretions also control the activities of entire systems of other glands. Their health and activity are considered vital to the health and activity of the entire body. And, while there are no studies that can show a direct relationship between these glands and arthritis, the lack of such studies might conceivably be the reason that no specific cause for arthritis has yet been discovered.

Certainly we have the subjective evidence of many thousands of arthritics who have benefited from exposure to sunlight. And for the first time we now have a rational explanation for the fact that many thousands of others have received absolutely no benefit from long periods of baking in the sun. While exposing their bodies, they may have been shielding their eyes with sunglasses and thus actually preventing the benefits they might have received if they had gone about fully clothed, but without any glass between their eyes and sunlight.

Even more to the point, those who wish relief may well have to go to the beaches for it because only at the shore are there clean breezes off the ocean with air clear enough for the sunlight to play its healing role. "Life on earth evolved under the full spectrum of natural sunlight, ranging from short ultraviolet wave lengths on one end to long infrared rays on the other," says Ott. "Too much of either extreme is harmful, but certain amounts of both are essential." He points out that window glass and indeed any type of glass will block out up to 99 percent of the ultraviolet light. This means that not only sunglasses, but also ordinary clear eyeglasses, will keep the eyes from receiving the potential benefits of the full spectrum of sunlight.

Believing completely that exposure of the eyes to sunlight is indispensable to full health in many aspects, including the retardation of aging, Dr. Ott, who now heads the Environmental Health and Light Research Institute in Sarasota, has developed new techniques of using plastics that transmit a full range of light for lenses, windows and special indoor lamps. In dealing with sunlight, however, it is necessary to sound some cautions.

To quote Dr. Ott in a *New Scientist* article (February 4, 1965), "Skin cancer is thought by many to be directly associated with excessive exposure to sunlight, and it is generally acknowledged that it is the ultraviolet part of the spectrum that is to blame. A number of different ailments of the eye are also related to excessive exposure to ultraviolet in sunlight." Sunlight is powerful. Be very cautious about it. Never look directly into the sun. It is in no way necessary to your efforts to ease the pain of arthritis. Indirect and reflected sunlight are just as good—perhaps better—so long as there is nothing actually preventing the ultraviolet rays from entering the eye.

In order to gain the possible benefits of sunlight entering the eye, it is not necessary to expose the skin of the body. Sunlight on the body in small, reasonable amounts activates vitamin D and improves health. But the amounts must be small. An excess *can* stimulate or cause skin cancer. Doctors recommend that you never expose yourself to enough sunlight to cause painful burning. Any discomfort associated with the exposure means you are getting too much.

However, the dangers of sun exposure may not be as great as

they used to be. I am sure many readers have noticed, as I have, that taking off your shirt while you mow the lawn for an hour just doesn't produce the sunburn that it used to. I have fair, sensitive skin, and twenty years ago I didn't dare uncover it on a city lawn for more than half an hour. Today I can spend several hours in shorts in my backyard and feel no effect. The difference, I am certain, lies in what the cement plants, automobiles and steel mills of the region are putting into the air.

If Dr. John Ott is right about what the lack of full-range light will do, the mounting pollution should be producing more arthritis. Statistics would bear this out. In 1961, according to government figures, there were 11,573,000 people in the United States receiving medical care for arthritis. In 1971, there were 17,000,-000. The increase is 48 percent, far outstripping the increase in population over the same period. Moreover, the Arthritis Foundation estimates that there are actually 50,000,000 people today—a full quarter of the population—who are to some extent arthritic.

I think the figures are significant and I personally believe there is a connection between the rising incidence of arthritis and polluted air. I do not think that inadequate light to the glands behind the eyes is the entire story, by any means. A few mummies from ancient Egypt have been found with evidence of arthritis, and the Egyptians surely lived in strong, clear sunshine. However, the complexity of bodily functions affected by the two glands involved—the pituitary, which is the body's master gland, and the pineal, which affects the functioning of the pituitary—is almost beyond imagining. The more they are studied, the more apparent it becomes that they affect just about everything we do and are. It is entirely believable that when functioning in a completely healthy way the glands would act to correct whatever metabolic defect induces arthritis, but fail to do so without the proper stimulation.

Nor is arthritis the only condition to be expected from malfunction of these light-sensitive glands. Let me list just a few of the ways in which it has been discovered we react to changes in light.

The most striking and widely-reported effects are on the human reproductive system. During the long Arctic night, Eskimo women do not menstruate and are in fact infertile. In general, people who live in the northern regions of the world experience a drop in sexual drive during the dark winter months. Children in the torrid zone mature sexually much earlier than their peers in more northerly countries. The effect of light on sex was graphically demonstrated by Dr. Richard Wurtman, an endocrinologist at the Massachusetts Institute of Technology. When he kept rats under fluorescent lighting, gonad, or sex gland, growth was retarded. But when the animals were kept under a full-spectrum light that mimics sunshine, the sex glands grew at a normal rate (*Endocrinology*, 85:1218–1221, 1969).

The color or wavelength of light also appears to be important in the bodily processes, Dr. Fritz Hollwich of the Münster University Eye Clinic in Germany told the New York Academy of Sciences at a special conference in 1963. Since then, Professor Hollwich has intensified his studies on the influence of light and with his colleague Professor Bernhard Dieckhues wrote an article for the journal *Fortschritte der Medizin* in which he cited an astonishing array of ways in which light affects physical functioning.

It begins at birth. Babies who are born blind lag behind those with normal sight in both growth and development. This is due, Hollwich and Dieckhues point out, to the delay in development of the pituitary gland caused by lack of light.

The pituitary influences the activities of many other glands. Therefore, it is not surprising that, even in adults, a lack of light is first noticed in the physical functions controlled by hormones. It was found that at the end of a long winter in limited light, members of a polar expedition suffered a number of illnesses. Their potency and sexual drive had decreased; their blood-sugar levels were lowered; their blood pressure was reduced; their hair tended to thin and they suffered from depression.

The researchers from Münster showed that a lack of light caused a pathological rise in the number of certain white corpuscles whereas light accelerated blood regeneration in cases of anemia.

A striking phenomenon was discovered by Hollwich and Dieckhues when the effect of light on urination was studied. A shortage of light, it seems, slows down the excretion of urine. Blind people, the researchers note, often look bloated because of the amount of water retained by their bodies. The flickering of normal fluorescent lighting increases urination, a fact of great importance for the staffs of most department stores and offices. The professors fear that too much artificial light could harm children and they advise strongly against building windowless schools.

The pituitary controls the body's lesser glands—the adrenals, the sex glands, the thyroid. The light messages getting through can determine whether the hormone production of the pituitary gland is normal. Therefore, light can profoundly influence many aspects of growth and health.

A research team headed by Dr. R. P. Feller reported an astonishing effect of sunlight on tooth decay at the March, 1970, meeting of the International Association for Dental Research. In an experiment, animals fed a high-sugar diet developed five times as many cavities when kept twelve hours a day under ordinary cool-white fluorescent lights as did control animals exposed to a fluorescent tube that approximated natural daylight. Of the thirty animals studied, the fifteen under natural-type fluorescent light averaged 2.2 cavities, compared to a 10.9 average in the group under ordinary fluorescent light.

Dr. Wurtman of MIT and his colleague Dr. Robert Neer examined the effects on calcium absorption of a white-light source whose emissions simulate the solar spectrum and found that living under such lighting for as little as five weeks enhances the intestinal absorption of calcium in healthy people (*New England Journal of Medicine,* February 17, 1970). By minimizing skin exposure to the full-spectrum light, the experimenters ruled out the possibility that vitamin D synthesis might have been responsible and established that it was indeed light passing through the eye that improved calcium absorption. And that might well be the key to the effect of light on arthritis, which is believed by many to result from calcium deficiency.

All right. Let's suppose that by now you are convinced, as I am, that we can all gain valuable health protection simply by getting more full-spectrum light into our eyes every day. What can you do about it?

If you wear eyeglasses, there are some brands of plastic lenses that transmit ultraviolet light, instead of screening it out as glass and most plastics do. Your optician ought to know about them.

The air is not yet contaminated enough to utterly filter out the wavelengths of light beyond the violet. It only reduces the amount of ultraviolet we receive. John Ott believes we ought to be able to compensate for this by receiving it for a longer period of time each day. He recommends that you spend more time outdoors, and that when you are outside, you either keep your glasses off or, if that is impossible, wear glasses made of an ultraviolet-transmitting plastic.

Suppose you can't, however? Suppose, like me, you do indoor work and have to keep at it during the daylight hours? John Ott has thought of that too, and being a superb technician, has done something about it. He has developed a fluorescent light that, used in your office's normal ceiling fixture, will provide both good illumination and that portion of the ultraviolet spectrum he has found experimentally will stimulate the pituitary and pineal glands. It will not burn or give you a synthetic suntan. The wavelengths with that effect are extraneous to the purpose and have been deliberately excluded.

What your eyes receive from these lights, beside illumination, is the same invisible ultraviolet light you would be getting sitting under a shade tree on a sunny day. The lights are already on the market. I use them in my office. And, as I write this, it occurs to me that a recurrent pain and stiffness in my right hip and a chronic feeling of weakness in the same area—as if I were always on the verge of a disabling attack and had to be careful how I put my feet down—have both disappeared. I just haven't had any such problem for the past couple of months, accepting the improvement without even thinking about it until this minute, when I have started wondering whether the light is responsible.

If you use the full-spectrum lights in your home or office, the light still won't get through the wrong kind of glasses. At the very least, take your glasses off for ten or fifteen minutes every now and then, and without looking directly at the light, which is unnecessary, let it bathe your eyes.

Finally, if sun glare hurts your eyes and you need sunglasses, a gray plastic lens will reduce the intensity of the entire spectrum, but totally eliminate none of it. Any other color will filter out the entire ultraviolet.

7   Treated Water Is No Treat

Whether we live in large or small cities, in suburban towns or on prairie farms, there are few of us indeed whose homes are not hooked into the municipal water supply. It is a great advantage, inevitably resulting in higher tax assessments, but a higher market value as well. Everyone knows that water—even the ground water that runs into wells—is polluted today and that drinking untreated water is a mild form of Russian roulette. We want our city water and we're willing to pay for it. Rightly so.

Only we wish it didn't have to taste so bad.

We hate the odor of chlorine and we hate its taste, but whether we complain or simply resign ourselves, we all know vaguely that the foul stuff is necessary to purify the water. And it is. Unless and until an equally effective substitute is found, chlorine is more necessary than most of us know.

It protects us against typhoid fever. It is, in fact, the simple, inexpensive public-health measure that has just about wiped out typhoid.

Typhoid comes from human excrement. And people in general are so strongly lacking in imagination and concern for social consequences that literally thousands of towns do not hesitate to flush their raw, untreated sewage right into the lakes and rivers that make up our supply of drinking water. They do it carefully, of course. They know which way the current runs and so Hiramville always runs its sewage pipes into the river at a point where the sewage will never return to Hiramville but will flow away to the next town down the line. Of course, Hiramville gets the load of the next town upstream in exchange.

Yes, it's illegal. And because they are inspected, the larger cities, which used to dispose of their wastes in the same cheap way, now treat and sanitize them before dumping them into the water. Smaller communities tend to feel they can't afford the "luxury." Even after receiving federal funding for sewage-treatment plants, a number of communities have been caught running untreated sewage into the river at night, while treating a portion of their wastes in the daytime.

There may be dispute about how much untreated sewage gets into drinking water these days, but I doubt that anyone would deny that chlorine—which kills the bacteria in human excrement that cause typhoid—is as necessary as ever in the treatment of drinking water. That is probably why nobody questions the use of chlorine, which is, after all, a poison gas. Like some other poisons, ionized chlorine plays a role in human nutrition, but one that is more than fulfilled by our use of common table salt— sodium chloride. How much more chlorine can you put into your body without ill effects? Well, your bottle of Clorox is labeled with stern warnings against drinking it or even getting it on your skin.

Where is the dividing line? How does daily drinking of chlorinated water affect human health? Even while we are being protected against deadly disease, is it possible that we are being harmed in other ways?

You may be amazed to learn that there has never been an organized, thorough investigation of the effect of chlorinated water on human—or even animal—health. There have been reports of allergic reactions—hives, asthma and functional colitis, among others. But no one has ever taken the trouble to compare a city of 100,000 people using chlorinated water with another of the same size whose water is not chlorinated to analyze differences in illness over a period of thirty or forty years.

Why not?

One good explanation may be fear of what might be learned. Because there is at least one competent physician—Dr. Joseph M. Price of Saginaw, Michigan—who has made his own extensive studies and concluded that chlorinated water causes heart disease. It is not a conclusion that has been generally accepted. But neither has it been investigated. In fact, it has been ignored.

What, after all, would happen if there were general agreement that the very same additive to drinking water that protects us from typhoid and other diseases—*and for which we have no substitute*—is at the same time a dangerous pollutant causing diseased arteries and heart attacks? Think of the turmoil. Think of the attacks on all the city governments and associations of water engineers and chemical manufacturers and users of chlorinated water in food processing. Think of the panic!

No wonder nobody wants to stick his neck out, or even look into the question, for fear he might reach conclusions that would force him to stick his neck out. Yet I think we have a right to know the evidence on which Dr. Price has based his conviction, to decide for ourselves how much merit it may have, and if we feel it's necessary, take steps to protect ourselves. The evidence is found in a book, *Coronaries, Cholesterol, Chlorine,* that Price has published with full-color illustrations.

The glossy color photos are intriguing, the story behind them even more so. They show row after row of chicken aortas, laid out on a clean, white surface. Some of them—cut open for closer examination—are pink and healthy, but others are bloated and covered with yellowish growths. These lumps don't belong in the chickens' blood vessels; they are fatty deposits—telltale signs of advanced atherosclerosis. Yet all the chickens were raised under identical conditions except for one factor: the diseased animals had chlorine added to their drinking water and feed.

For his study, Dr. Price selected one hundred day-old cockerels. (The male chicken, like the male human being, is more susceptible to the development of atherosclerosis.) The methodology and results are described by the author:

Both groups were placed on a cooked mash consisting of about a 1:1 mixture of corn and oat meals with about 5 per cent low-priced oleomargarine added. Pure distilled water was used exclusively. Chlorine was added to the drinking water and mash of the experimental group in the form of chlorine bleach (disinfectant), about one-third teaspoonful per quart of water. This highly chlorinated water was first given to the experimental group at twelve weeks of age.

The results were nothing short of spectacular! Within three weeks there were grossly observable effects on both appearance and behavior. The experimental group became lethargic, huddling in corners except at feeding time. Their feathers became frayed and dirty and the cockerels walked around with their wings hunched up, their feathers fluffed up like they were always cold (the experiment was performed in an unheated barn in winter), their pale combs drooping. This appearance is most suggestive of symptoms resulting from clogging up of the micro-circulation.

The control group, on the other hand, was observed to thrive. Chickens not ingesting chlorine were larger in size and more active, with clean, shiny feathers. But, as Dr. Price was to discover, the contrast was more than skin deep.

"No less remarkable was the gross appearance of the aortas," he notes.

The abdominal aortas [the place where atherosclerosis is known to occur in chickens] of all of the cockerels dying after four months were carefully examined. In more than 95 per cent of the experimental group grossly visible thick yellow plaques of atherosclerosis protruding into the lumens were discovered! These chickens were noted to have an extremely high apparently spontaneous death rate and common findings on examination of the carcasses were hemorrhage into the lungs and enlarged hearts.

After seven months, he says, *every chicken* fed chlorinated water had developed atherosclerosis, while *not a single chicken* of the pure-water control group had done so. When a check was made by feeding chlorinated water to the control cockerels, they too developed atherosclerotic lesions.

What led Dr. Price to experiment with chlorine in the first place? He was puzzled by the fantastic surge in the incidence of heart disease (heart attack, stroke, atherosclerosis) during this century. Noting that prior to 1900 such cases were almost unheard of, he reasoned "that something has changed in the last 6–7 decades of human history."

It is a fact that Dr. Paul Dudley White, a leading cardiologist, has written that he did not see his first heart attack of the type caused by atherosclerosis until after 1920. He had not seen any as a student and intern. In 1910, when the great physician Sir William Osler published his lectures on heart disease, he didn't mention this type of heart attack—and it is now the leading cause of death in the United States.

Price was fascinated by evidence that heart attacks, while occurring before 1930, only reached proportions significant enough to affect mortality statistical tables at that time. He suspected that some environmental factor, crucial to the development of atherosclerosis, was being overlooked by medical science.

Experimental use of chlorine to "purify" water supplies began in the late 1890's [he points out]. Chlorination gained relatively wide acceptance in the second decade of this century and in the third decade (1920's) it was found that satisfactory killing of organisms was dependent upon a *residual* of chlorine in the water above the amount necessary to react with organic impurities. When it is remembered that evidence of clinical disease from atherosclerosis takes 10–20 years to develop, it becomes evident that there is a correlation between the introduction and widespread application of chlorination of water supplies and the origin and increasing incidence of heart attacks that is exceedingly difficult to explain away.

To back up his argument, the author brings in evidence from

around the globe: Japan has a low incidence of heart attack, but when Japanese move to Hawaii and drink chlorinated water, they develop atherosclerosis. Some Africans eat a very high-cholesterol diet but drink no chlorinated water—and they don't get heart attacks. Irish farm workers studied by Dr. Paul Dudley White, who drink their own well water, *never* develop coronary heart disease.

Finally, Dr. Price observes that during the Korean War autopsies performed on young American soldiers killed in battle revealed over 75 percent showed evidence of coronary atherosclerosis although their average age was only 22.1 years. Although most medical men took this as surprising evidence of the early onslaught of so-called degenerative disease, the author offers a different explanation:

> If you ask any man who served in that war he will tell you that the water in Korea for our soldiers was so heavily chlorinated for sanitary reasons that it was almost undrinkable. . . . Apparently, there is a direct *causal* correlation between the amount of chlorine ingested and the speed and degree of development of atherosclerosis!

For statistical comparison, in 1900 before chlorination was in very general use, there were 35,379 deaths from typhoid in the United States, or about 31 per 100,000 of population. In that same year, 1900, there were 68,439 deaths from heart disease, or 137 per 100,000 of population. By 1950, as a result of the use of chlorine, plus a general improvement in the sanitation of the water supply, there were only 90 deaths from typhoid in the United States, which means that it is now down to practically zero. But heart disease by 1950 had skyrocketed up to 535,930 deaths or 355 per 100,000 of population. The effect of chlorine? Price believes so.

In 1969, Professor Joshua Lederberg, a Stanford University biochemist and Nobel laureate, pointed out in his syndicated newspaper column that when water chlorination was first introduced sixty years ago, tests made at that time to show it nontoxic were laughable by modern scientific standards. He went on to show that "almost no attention has been given to the subject of chronic toxicity from chlorine." He added,

We have no clear picture of the place, manner, intermediate products or rate by which chlorine (poison gas) is converted into chloride ion (safe) within the body. . . . What little we do know of the chemistry of chlorine reactions is portentous.

The reactions of chlorine with DNA have been remarkably little studied. In my own search in the literature, I found only a single oblique reference. Chlorine . . . rapidly inactivated DNA that had been isolated from bacteria.

We know little more of the mechanism by which chlorine kills bacteria. The scanty data suggests that the most likely mechanism is precisely by attack on the DNA of the microbe.

DNA, of course, is nucleic acid, the material containing the programmed instructions for the size, shape and function of every cell of our bodies. Anything that can injure DNA is, at least potentially, a major menace.

Perhaps it was Professor Lederberg's urging that struck a spark, not among American scientists, but in Japan. Two years after his column appeared, a study by Professor Ukita and his associates of the faculty of pharmaceutical sciences at the University of Tokyo was published in the *Chemical Pharmaceutical Bulletin*. This paper reported the first study of the effect of chlorine on nucleic acids and also on their constituents, those materials that the body uses to manufacture nucleic acids. And what the Japanese scientists found was that, beyond a doubt, chlorine does chemically alter the nucleic acids, although the significance of this to human health can only be guessed at thus far.

The first effect was that in reaction to chlorine the color of both DNA and transfer RNA was changed, so that both types of nucleic acids became more opaque and therefore less able to absorb ultraviolet light. Whether this is of any significance to health would be very hard to say, although it is much safer to assume that anything that alters the nucleic acids in any way will also induce changes in their function. And any change in nucleic-acid function must induce what by definition is an abnormality, even though it may be a slight one.

Let me give you an example to make this a little clearer. You cut your hand with a bread knife and, after it bleeds a while, the blood clots and closes the wound. Then the wound heals. How? The cells in the region of the wound are somehow instructed by the nucleic acids to reproduce themselves and replace those cells that have been killed or injured by the cut. When the wound has been closed by new living tissue, the cells must then be instructed to stop their fast growth and reproduction. It all works like a charm, and when we say that the wound has healed, we mean that it is no longer open and just the right amounts of muscle and epithelial tissue have been replaced in the right places. But obviously any change whatsoever from the normal in the nucleic acids can make some kind of change in the instructions that they issue. If they no longer tell the cells when to stop their rapid reproduction, then there is going to be an abnormal growth at the site of the wound. Or perhaps the wound won't heal at all. Or perhaps scar tissue will not form where it is needed. Or perhaps the new skin will lack pigmentation. No matter what the abnormality, it is undesirable.

There is another possibility, however, which is that nucleic acid that has been damaged by chlorine will itself be replaced with new undamaged nucleic acid. And it must be supposed that a great deal of this goes on, since practically all of us drink chlorinated water and yet we are not continually producing abnormalities.

But the Japanese scientists found that chlorine also affects the precursors of nucleic acids, a group of chemicals with such names as thymine, uracil, adenosine and guanine. And it is very hard to believe that damaged precursors could be formed into healthy nucleic acid.

So we get a picture of the admittedly small amount of chlorine we drink doing some damage to our nucleic acid and its precursors, perhaps involving our bodies in a continual struggle to keep replacing these damaged vital materials. Can this be related to the observable fact that as our bodies get older and can only synthesize new nucleic acid at a slower rate, the number of surface and internal abnormalities we develop increases sharply? The answer is yes, according to "Potential Carcinogenicity of Sodium Hypochloride," a paper published in *Nature* (October 15, 1971) and written by scientists from the National Cancer Center Research Institute in Tokyo. Sodium hypochloride is the form in which chlorine is added to water, and the paper claims that chlorine is a co-carcinogen. In other words, it says that chlorine will not cause cancer itself, but that it will reinforce the effect and make more virulent the stimulation of cancer by other materials. So it begins to look as though Professor Lederberg may have been right in pointing out that the safety of chlorine has not been demonstrated at all by modern standards, and that it should be investigated thoroughly.

The Japanese have even produced laboratory confirmation of Dr. Price's claim that chlorine induces atherosclerosis. In the pharmaceutical laboratories of the University of Tokyo a team of investigators examined the effect on human blood cells of chlorinated city water, and found that some of the red cells of the blood are destroyed by such water. This in itself is no major problem. Red cells are always dying and being replaced anyway. But they also found that chlorinated water increases the tendency of the cells of the blood to clump together. This agglutination, leading to the formation of clots of blood cells within the arteries, is one of the key elements in the condition known as atherosclerosis.

Is chlorine a cause of atherosclerosis? If so, is it a major or minor cause? If it is a threat to health, how much does it take to do the damage? These questions deserve more consideration than they are getting. Nor do I pretend to have any hard answers. What

I do know beyond a doubt is that chlorine in my tap water is obnoxious stuff. It smells bad and tastes bad. It does not improve the flavor of my coffee and what it does to tea is a sin.

I don't know any way to eliminate it at the waterworks, but with a little trouble I can improve the situation in my own home. So can you. If you boil water for three minutes, you will remove 65 to 70 percent of the chlorine it contains, which will greatly improve its taste and odor, and render it safer as well. Remember that neither Dr. Price nor anyone else would suggest that you try to eliminate all chlorine from your diet. It is the excess he considers dangerous, and cutting down by 65 percent on the amount you receive from water should greatly improve the situation.

If you decide to do it, the simplest way is to estimate how much water your family uses in a day, and boil up that much in the morning, if you have the time, or at night before you go to bed. As soon as it's cool enough, pour it into glass containers—milk bottles are fine—and store them in the refrigerator if you have the room. Otherwise, it won't do any harm to let the water stand on a counter, as long as the glass container is full and its top closed. That is just about the equivalent of letting it stand in the water pipe. Note that three minutes of boiling is enough. Boiling for a longer time will not remove any more of the chlorine.

It is also possible, if you own your own home, to get chlorine-free water at the tap by installing a charcoal filter in the basement. Unfortunately, it costs quite a bit, but it does save trouble, and it does work, if you can afford it.

I consider boiling preferable, on the whole, since it not only removes a good portion of the chlorine, but also kills other bacteria on which chlorine has no effect—and most water can surely use this extra sterilization. Boiling also leaves most of the mineral content of the water intact, and it is the minerals that give water its flavor. Filtered water sometimes tastes flat.

8 Can Tap Water Hurt Linus Pauling?

One pollutant you cannot boil out of your tap water is nitrate, which is generally recognized as dangerous. Since no municipal water-treatment plant will make any effort to remove it, you will have to take steps to protect yourself. This, fortunately, you can do.

That this important safety measure should be left to you is a tribute to the talent of government health agencies for basing their regulations on obsolete information. In the case of water quality it is the Public Health Service that sets the standards, and the Public Health Service has decided that water may safely contain up to forty-five parts per million of nitrate.

The PHS determination is based upon medical information about how much nitrate it takes to induce a rare and infrequently fatal blood disease, methemoglobinemia, in infants. Fifteen years ago that was, indeed, the only disease that was known to be caused by a high nitrate content in water.

Since that time, however, there has accumulated a mountain of evidence that nitrate is an estimable potential cause of cancer in the gastrointestinal tract, that it has probably killed many people already, and that it is going to kill many more. Official notice of this more recent information, however, has not yet been taken, and forty-five parts per million remains the official permissible level of nitrate in drinking water. At any concentration below that level, water is considered officially safe, and no effort is made to remove the nitrate.

So how do I know that there's nitrate in your water, whether you live in New York, New Orleans or Goshen, Indiana?

Because it's everywhere.

Nitrate is an essential plant food. It is created in nature by bacteria in the soil, which convert nitrogen from the air into small amounts of stable nitrate in the ground. The nitrate is absorbed by plants that use it for growth. So far, so good.

But, when it comes to commercial farming, the amount of nitrate naturally fixed in the soil doesn't begin to be adequate to produce the quantity of food per acre that farmers want. So the farmers spread, over billions of acres of farmland, chemical fertilizers with a much higher nitrate content than anything nature ever produced. These fertilizers are designed to give the plants all the nitrate they can use, and then some. Even after a growing season has ended, there is always a high nitrate residue lying right on the surface of our farmland from coast to coast.

Along come the winter snows, followed by the spring thaw and a heavy runoff of water into streams. The runoff contains nitrate in large amounts. The streams run into the rivers and eventually the same water gets to your tap, still loaded with nitrate. Actually, this process doesn't require a winter of heavy snow. A single heavy rain will have the same effect.

In *The Closing Circle* Barry Commoner describes a study he made of Decatur, Illinois, and refers to "data from the Illinois State Water Survey, which shows that between 1958 and 1965, when nitrogen fertilizer use increased fourfold, the nitrate levels of a number of the rivers that drain Illinois farmlands increased significantly. There was good reason to believe that the intensive use of nitrogen fertilizer was the basic cause of the dangerously high levels of nitrate in the Decatur water supply."

Chemical nitrates aren't the only source of trouble. Animal manure also contains generous amounts of nitrate, which is one reason why manure is an excellent fertilizer when it's spread out on fields. But today, the agricultural landscape is punctuated—and polluted—with mind-and-nose-boggling heaps of cattle, swine and poultry waste. Produced in superefficient feedlots, batteries, and other prisonlike compounds, these waste piles release fantastic amounts of concentrated nitrate into local streams and then into rivers every time it rains. Or they may leach nitrates through the soil into underground water tables. Nitrate-rich animal tankage, the waste product of slaughterhouses, is often dumped by the ton into rivers, because with all the cheap and superpowerful chemical fertilizers around, few farmers want the tankage for their fields, no matter how good it is for soil health. And, of course, don't forget human sewage, millions of tons of which winds up in rivers every day, further adding to the nitrate burden of drinking and irrigation water.

Yet all of this nitrate piling up in our drinking water might not be too dangerous except for some biochemical transformations that take place both in and out of our bodies. The commonest transformation results from bacterial action that changes nitrate into a chemically similar but much more dangerous form called nitrite.

Nitrite is so poisonous that it is used as a preservative in food, permitted because it will kill the bacteria that produce botulism. But, because it is so highly toxic, it is permitted to be added to food only in tiny quantities. Still, food technologists value it highly, because it also has a fabulous ability to keep meat red. For this purpose alone, nitrite is added to some eight billion pounds a year of hot dogs, other sausages and canned hams.

And, since they are permitted to use only a little bit of it, the technologists take advantage of precisely the same transformation that menaces us. They add to the same meat much larger amounts of the relatively innocuous nitrate, and rely on the bacteria present to transform it into nitrite while it is being stored. That is why hot dogs stay red for weeks.

What happens, tests have shown, is that the bacteria normally found in meat work on the nitrate and reduce it to nitrite. And it's the nitrite that does the cosmetic and preservative work. Many processors use some nitrate as a sort of nitrite time-release capsule. The label on the lunch meat may say "sodium nitrate added" but you can be sure that, by the time you eat it, much or all of the nitrate has been transformed into nitrite.

The bacteria that perform this service for the meat processors are hardly scarce. They're known as nitrate-reducing bacteria and are found nearly everywhere.

One place these bacteria call home is the leaves of spinach and other green vegetables. But they don't go to work until after the spinach has been picked, so if you eat spinach picked fresh from your garden, there is no reason to be concerned. But, if you eat spinach that has been shipped for some distance and then stored in warehouses or supermarket counters, you can be sure that a substantial amount of nitrate has been turned into nitrite by bacteria (A. Sinios and W. Wodsak, *Deutsches Medizinische Wochenschrift,* 90; 1965). The longer your vegetables have been stored before you eat them, the more nitrite they contain.

These nitrate reducers also thrive in the human body, and can begin changing nitrates into nitrites within moments of entering the system. This is especially and tragically true in infants, as a result of their weak stomach acidity. Given a bottleful of water sufficiently polluted with nitrate to work on, the bacteria in the baby's stomach turn out nitrites so abundantly that they combine chemically with red blood cells and render them incapable of carrying oxygen. This condition, called methemoglobinemia, mentioned earlier, turns the baby blue and can chemically suffocate it. According to a special report by the American Chemical Society in 1969, *Cleaning Our Environment,* "from 1947 to 1950, Minnesota alone reported 139 cases of methemoglobinemia, including 14 deaths, caused by nitrate in farm water."

For many years, it was thought that this transformation could take place only in the stomach of an infant less than five months or so old. But recently evidence has been published that this is not the case. Dr. Johannes Sander of West Germany, according to an editorial in the *Journal of the American Medical Association* (May 17, 1971), has shown experimentally that adult stomachs can also reduce nitrate to nitrite if acidity is low, as it is in many people most of the time, and in most people toward the end of a meal. The sheer size of adults, however, precludes the kind of acute reaction that can sometimes swiftly kill infants.

Now that we understand how nitrite reaches our stomachs, we must be perfectly honest and state that nitrite as such isn't what cancer and public-health specialists are worrying about—except for contamination of well water and the subsequent deadly threat to babies. True, some adults have been fatally poisoned by eating foods containing excessive amounts of nitrite. Cases are described by Berton Roueche in *Eleven Blue Men* (Little, Brown, Boston, 1954). But there is another danger involving nitrite in our stomachs which is of far greater concern to these scientists—and should be to you, too.

That fear is that nitrite, once in the stomach, combines with substances called *secondary amines* to form compounds known as *nitrosamines*. Nitrosamines are known to cause cancer. All that is necessary to trigger this reaction is for nitrite and a secondary amine to be present together in the stomach. A process called *nitrosation* takes place, resulting in the formation of the cancer-causing nitrosamines.

Dr. William Lijinsky and Dr. Samuel Epstein, in a study published in *Nature* (January 3, 1970), cite literature showing that various nitrosamines fed to animals produce cancer of the esophagus, stomach and lungs. The *Journal of the National Cancer Institute* (48; 1972) abstracted the most recent test results reported by Dr. Sidney S. Mirvish and others at the Eppley Institute for Research in Cancer, University of Nebraska Medical Center, Omaha, which demonstrate, quite plainly, that nitrite and amines fed to a mouse at the same time also result in lung tumors (as many as ten times more than in control animals), and overwhelm the liver with toxins. It was reported in the *New York Times* (July 12, 1972) that the International Agency for Research on Cancer, in Lyons, France, has identified nitrite compounds as "one of the prime suspects" in cancer of the esophagus.

These studies, along with test-tube procedures and a knowledge of human stomach chemistry, have convinced most researchers that there is no known reason why this same process of nitrosation would not take place in a human stomach when nitrites and secondary amines come together.

By now we know where nitrites come from; what about the secondary amines? According to Lijinsky and Epstein, you are eating large amounts of these amines when you eat any kind of fish, especially salt-water fish. Do you have cereal for breakfast? You are eating secondary amines. Do you enjoy a cup of tea? You are enjoying secondary amines. Have you ever sat next to a person who was smoking? You were inhaling his secondary amines along with his smoke. And, if you have ever taken any one of a rather large number of drugs, you were also taking secondary amines.

Dr. Moizo Ishidate, director of the Tokyo Biochemical Research Institute, was quoted in *Medical Tribune* (March 22, 1972) as singling out powdered milk and sausage as foods especially high in nitrosatable amines. He also points out that cooked or processed foods tend to be higher in secondary amines than raw foods. Other researchers have named various grains, as well as alcoholic beverages made from these grains, as sources of amines.

Clearly, it would be just as difficult to design a diet free of secondary amines as it would be to choose one free of all nitrates. It would be almost as difficult never to eat the two together in an attempt to block nitrosation. You would never be able to eat vegetables with any kind of bread, grain or fish; never drink tea at the end of a meal; and never so much as sip a glass of wine if anyone at the table was smoking a cigarette.

You are probably thinking, in that case, why doesn't *everyone* have cancer?

Well, that is the very question which many researchers in various parts of the world are asking themselves. They are probing their statistics, examining small differences in regional diets. Dr. Sander, previously mentioned, says there is a link between weak stomach acidity and cancer of the stomach. The weak acidity could permit a much higher production of nitrites, as occurs in babies. Any one or many of an infinite number of metabolic differences could also enter the picture. One difference that has come to seem increasingly important is the amount of vitamin C in the stomach.

New experimental data showing that vitamin C can chemically smash nitrites and prevent the formation of nitrosamines comes from four cancer specialists at the Eppley Institute for Research in Cancer.

The scientists—Dr. Sidney S. Mirvish, Dr. Lawrence Wallcave, Dr. Michael Eagen and Dr. Phillippe Shubik—were so impressed with the potency of small amounts of ascorbic acid (vitamin C) in destroying nitrites that they recommend in their papers in *Science* (July 7, 1972) that the vitamin be routinely taken as a precautionary measure whenever any one of a large number of foods or drugs that could combine with the nitrites into nitrosamines are ingested. That way, nitrites are wiped out in the stomach before they have a chance to cause any mischief.

These researchers combined nitrite with various secondary amines under varying conditions of acidity which had already been shown to produce nitrosamines. But when they added vitamin C to the brew, and analyzed the contents, they discovered that, on the average, the process of nitrosation had been blocked about 97 to 99 percent!

In one case, though, there was more nitrosation, but only under conditions of extreme acidity. In all likelihood, the nitrite in the food would be destroyed before the food reached that point of acidity.

Mr. Mirvish and his colleagues mention eight drugs among those known to contain secondary amines. If they were taken just before some nitrited fish or hot dogs or even with water containing a high burden of nitrates, the stage would be set for nitrosation and the production of nitrosamines. Therefore, they urge the medical-scientific community, doesn't it make sense to prescribe a small amount of vitamin C to be taken with every pill? They also suggest that vitamin C be added to any food product which contains nitrates or nitrites, as a preventive measure. Why gamble with cancer when prevention is so simple and so inexpensive?

As yet, however, no food manufacturers have leaped to accept the invitation. Not because of the cost—the vitamin is pathetically inexpensive—but more likely precisely because of the characteristics that are so protective in the gastrointestinal tract.

Vitamin C—ascorbic acid—is what is known chemically as a reducing agent. It will easily yield an electron to another chemical—in this case nitrite—that is composed in such a way as to welcome such intrusions. Unless the nitrite gets the electron from ascorbic acid first, it will try to get it from a secondary amine if one is present, forming, in the process, a carcinogenic nitrosamine. But the electron from ascorbic acid gets there faster and has a stabilizing effect, so that the nitrite is no longer a candidate for nitrosation.

Nor is it only nitrite that vitamin C renders immune to corruption. It has the same stabilizing hence detoxifying effect on literally hundreds of chemicals that find their way into our bodies, from the nicotine of cigarettes to the toxic products of virus infections.

If vitamin C were added to hot dogs, it would have much the same effect. It would prevent the nitrates from turning into nitrites—and instead of staying that repulsively unnatural red that customers demand, the hot dogs would turn brown. No self-respecting food technologist is going to sit still for that. If any manufacturer brought out a brown hot dog, such as we used to eat when I was a boy, and people bought it anyway, his next idea might be that he didn't need any technologists on his payroll.

So we can be pretty sure that those bright people who devote their lives to changing the color, flavor and texture of food will not hastily add half a cent's worth of vitamin C just to protect us from cancer. A couple of companies have announced that they are considering the addition, but they have not announced any date for implementation.

We may as well take our own.

How much? That's a good question.

Actually it would require remarkably little to counteract the small quantity of nitrite that reaches or is formed in our stomachs. Except? Well, it has to be there at precisely the same time to do any good, which means not only when you go to the company picnic but every time you drink a glass of water. Then it must be remembered that in parting with electrons to detoxify hundreds of substances, vitamin C literally destroys itself.

So if you want to be sure, let's say, that there are ten milligrams of the vitamin in your stomach every time you drink water, coffee or tea, or eat a food containing nitrites and/or nitrates, it becomes a question less of the potency of the tablet than of how often you take one.

Whether you take large or small doses, taking them frequently is good policy for a simple physiological reason. Vitamin C is an acid. The normal condition of the blood is slightly alkaline, and in working to maintain that condition, the kidneys filter the ascorbic acid out of the bloodstream. In about five hours, whatever vitamin C you have taken that has gotten into the blood serum has ended up in your urinary bladder. If you wait until next morning to get more, you will be going an appreciable time with none of the free vitamin circulating through your system. That, in the opinion of Linus Pauling, Irwin Stone and a rapidly growing group of medical believers in "megavitamins," would be a sad state of affairs. These leading scientists believe that almost without limit the more vitamin C we get, the better off we are.

Irwin Stone, the biochemist to whom Linus Pauling dedicated his book *Vitamin C and the Common Cold,* doesn't believe that vitamin C is a vitamin at all. And he doesn't believe that the vitamin-C-deficiency disease, scurvy, should be so classified or regarded as a nutritional disorder. In fact, he argues, the prevailing concept of ascorbic acid as "vitamin C" (which cures scurvy when given in trace amounts) is the single biggest reason why medical research has failed to test the therapeutic value of ascorbic acid given in massive doses—doses which are logically called for under a quite different concept of what ascorbic acid is all about.

In Stone's opinion, man's dietary need for ascorbic acid is a biological accident. And man's chronic shortage of ascorbic acid— a shortage which becomes extreme in the case of scurvy—is the consequence of a genetic disease, which Stone calls hypoascorbemia. We inherit hypoascorbemia from a remote primate ancestor who suffered the "biochemical catastrophe" of a mutation (an accidentally changed gene) which destroyed a liver enzyme necessary for ascorbic-acid synthesis. Almost all mammals possess this enzyme (L-gulonolactone oxidase) and manufacture their own ascorbic acid—and so did man's ancestor before the mutation took place, Stone believes.

Although the species became totally dependent on food for its ascorbic-acid needs, Stone says, it is nevertheless incorrect, biologically speaking, to define ascorbic acid as a nutrient or vitamin; rather it is a "missing endogenous product"—that is, a substance "normally" synthesized within the body.

In judging how much ascorbic acid is required for optimum human health, we should be guided by how much is synthesized by "normal" mammals, Stone says. He points out that nearly all mammals produce ascorbic acid plentifully, saturating blood and tissue, and—most importantly—stepping up production under conditions of stress when the body draws most heavily on its ascorbic-acid stores.

Stone suggests "correction" of man's genetic disease, hypoascorbemia, by ascorbic-acid intake in an amount comparable to that produced by other mammals—in other words, in the amount humans would be synthesizing for themselves had the genetic defect never occurred. These amounts are measured in grams—not the milligrams of the Food and Nutrition Board's "recommended daily allowance."

Infectious diseases, cardiovascular disorders, collagen diseases, cancer, and the aging process—these are some of the human ills, Stone says, that scanty evidence suggests might be unequivocally moderated by ascorbic acid given at the dosage level called for by the genetic concept. For conclusive evidence, he calls on the medical community to test his theory with widespread clinical studies.

Stone presents his ascorbic-acid thesis, with supporting evidence, in four published papers (*American Journal of Physical Anthropology,* March, 1965; *Perspectives in Biology and Medicine,* Autumn, 1966; and *Acta Geneticae Medicae et Gemellologiae,* October, 1966 and January, 1967). He has also published a book on the subject: *The Healing Factor* (Grosset and Dunlap, 1972).

In the mid-1930s, Stone developed for the research laboratory he directs the use of ascorbic acid as an antioxidant for food preservation—receiving a patent for the process, which is now widely in use. But it was the medical rather than the industrial use of ascorbic acid that fascinated him, sending him to haunt New York's medical libraries, comb and analyze research as reported in the medical literature, and eventually come to his conclusion that the vitamin C concept, with its presumptions about "trace" amounts, is all wrong.

Acting on his own convictions, Stone (and the rest of his family) began taking daily doses of ascorbic acid in large amounts, working up to between 3 and 5 grams daily (as compared with 70 milligrams in the "recommended daily allowance"). The size of the dose Stone calculated from the amount of ascorbic acid synthesized by the rat—equivalent to 4.9 grams a day for man and 15 grams under conditions of stress.

In 1960, when Stone was the victim of a near-fatal automobile accident, he upped his dosage to the even higher stress levels of thirty to forty grams a day and succeeded in leaving the hospital in three months instead of the full year predicted by his physician. Except for the accident, Stone comments, he has enjoyed vibrant health under his ascorbic-acid regimen and has suffered no illness, not even a common cold.

As to the potential "toxicity" of ascorbic acid in large doses—something which some conservative doctors are making a big thing about in opposition to Linus Pauling's book—Stone points to ascorbic acid's long documented record as "the least toxic of any known substance of comparable physiological activity." Furthermore, he elaborates, while human investigators have not tested the safety of large amounts of ascorbic acid taken over long periods of time, nature *has*.

"There is good evolutionary reason," he writes, "for [ascorbic acid's] complete lack of toxicity. Living organisms have been exposed to fairly high levels of ascorbic acid throughout eons of time, if this can be judged from its widespread occurrence in all forms of present day life from the simplest to the most complex. If ascorbic acid had any toxicity that would have been detrimental to survival, it would have been eliminated long ago by the evolutionary process."

Only a very few species throughout the entire animal and plant world have lost their ability to synthesize ascorbic acid. Among animals, only man and other higher primates, the guinea pig, an Indian fruit-eating bat, and a bird (the red-vented bulbul), are known to be dependent on food for their ascorbic acid needs and can contract and die of scurvy.

Since there are so few animals unable to manufacture ascorbic acid, many scientists believe that a past mutation is responsible in each case for this deviant physiology. Stone is not the author of a new theory in this respect. Where he offers a new insight is in seeing man as continuing to be disabled, handicapped, in fact, "diseased" by his ancestor's genetic accident.

We must presume that originally the mutation presented no problems to the species because of ample food stores of ascorbic acid in year-round vegetation. (A gorilla living in a tropical jungle habitat is estimated to consume about 4.5 grams of ascorbic acid in his daily enormous intake of vegetation.) In the case of man's ancestor, we must even presume that the mutated individuals had an actual survival advantage over their brothers whose liver enzyme, L-gulonolactone oxidase, remained intact—otherwise the latter group would have been the one to have survived to the twentieth century. Discussing this matter in his book, Linus Pauling points to geneticists' findings that there is a kind of biological "economy," with survival value in loss of a physiological function, provided the species can adjust to the change without disadvantage. (Our ancestor's adjustment, for example, might have been the inclusion for the first time of fruits and vegetables in the diet.)

But what happens when an advantageous situation changes?

"As soon as man or his primitive ancestors left their original tropical or semi-tropical environment and moved to the temperate climes where fresh vegetation was no longer available the year round, they were in trouble," Stone writes. And the dietary habits they developed only compounded their distress. "With the discovery of fire and the development of cooking, the fresh raw meat and fish of man's early diet which were fairly rich sources of exogenous ascorbic acid lost much of this vital substance because of its sensitivity to heat-enhanced oxidation. . . . Primitive agriculture with its emphasis on the easily storable cereal crops provided foodstuffs essentially devoid of any ascorbic acid."

Stone concludes: "It is mute testimony to the ruggedness and adaptability of the human organism that man was able to survive on such low levels of ascorbic acid compared with the amounts produced by other mammals. Survive he did, but the toll in disease, misery and death must have been great."

Scurvy has caused more deaths, Stone speculates, and created more human misery and has altered the course of human history more than any other single cause. For centuries scurvy has been associated with dietary needs. For the past half century, as the nutritional sciences and vitamin theory developed, the accepted explanation of scurvy is that it is a nutritional disorder caused by lack of the trace nutrient vitamin C in foodstuffs.

But the *true* cause of scurvy, Stone says (as well as of less obvious forms of ascorbic-acid deprivation) is the missing enzyme. Hypoascorbemia fits perfectly into the genetic-disease classification: "A disease caused by an inherited defect in the gene which controls the synthesis of the particular enzyme whose absence or lack of activity causes the specific pathologic metabolic syndrome."

As Stone observes, there is more to this contention than a fascinating concept or a mere matter of semantics: "The genetic concept provides a new rationale for the therapeutic use of high levels of ascorbic acid either alone or in combination with other medicaments, and opens vistas of clinical testing in many areas that have lain fallow in the decades since the discovery of ascorbic acid (1932)."

Stone's concept offers a fully rational explanation of how and why it should be that vitamin C has been found remarkably effective—often unexpectedly so—against a host of unrelated poisons. Fred Klenner, a North Carolina physician, has used it successfully against rattlesnake bite and as a general antibiotic, a treatment that has been confirmed by the Pasteur Institute in Paris. The vitamin has been used as a specific against fever and gastrointestinal disorders.

Recently the vitamin has emerged as a probable source of real protective value against cadmium, a little-known pollutant that Dr. Henry Schroeder, an expert on mineral nutrition, considers a major cause of high blood pressure. Dr. T. C. Hindson of Singapore gave vitamin C to children as young as four months to clear up severe prickly heat. The dose was 50 milligrams a day for a 7.5-pound baby, 100 milligrams a day for a 15-pound baby, etc. "No unwanted side effects appeared," he reported in *Lancet,* June 22, 1968. All the children were cured of their prickly heat.

The vitamin, when available, even saturates the leukocytes, the white cells of the blood that engulf and destroy invading bacteria. And a great deal of the ability of the leukocytes to protect against infection depends on the availability of vitamin C, according to a study by Dr. H. S. Loh and Dr. C. W. M. Wilson, titled "Relationship Between Leucocyte and Plasma Ascorbic Acid Concentrations," published in the *British Medical Journal,* September 25, 1971.

It therefore makes a lot of sense to take some vitamin C with every meal—and drink, too. If you have reason to believe the nitrate content of your drinking water is unusually high, it becomes urgent to protect any infant in your family with vitamin C. Add a small amount of vitamin C to his water, maybe one-third of a powdered 100-milligram tablet to a 4-ounce bottle. It doesn't take much vitamin C to knock out nitrite, and unless your water is terribly contaminated, this amount should provide protection.

So here is one more reason why we should not only take vitamin C and take it several times a day, but also take considerably more than government-sanctioned allowances, which are based only on the amount needed to prevent deficiency symptoms. As we've seen, vitamin C can do a great deal more than prevent scurvy.

Finally, if you're as sold on vitamin C as I am, you will certainly want to learn the recently revealed secret of one of the most important scientists in the history of the vitamin as to how to bring out the best in it.

The man is Albert Szent-Györgyi, the brilliant biochemist who first isolated ascorbic acid and proved it to be vitamin C, and who in 1937 was awarded the Nobel Prize for his studies of the metabolism of vitamins A and C. Throughout his life Dr. Szent-Györgyi has suffered with chronic colds, with pneumonia as an occasional aftermath. He is as interested as Linus Pauling in preventing colds with vitamin C and has gone a step further. He now includes in his daily diet a food that, by biochemical processes he describes in a recent book, *The Living State,* doubles, triples or even further multiplies the effectiveness of the vitamin. The food—wheat germ.

Dr. Szent-Györgyi, born in 1893, believes that he owes to this combination of wheat germ and vitamin C not only freedom from colds in his later years, but also the very fact that he has lived as long as he has. To which I might add that his life is not only long but that, at nearly eighty, his mind remains as active and fertile as it ever was and the brilliant discoveries he has already made may turn out to be only a prelude to what is yet to come from that extraordinary intelligence.

In his book Dr. Szent-Györgyi describes how, after the isolation of ascorbic acid in crystalline form in 1930, he became aware in the next year that there seemed to be some element missing that would permit ascorbic acid to function with regard to human respiration the same way that it does in plants. It took another thirty-five years for him to discover the missing element.

Sixteen years ago he began eating wheat germ, banana and milk for breakfast every day, also including 2,000 milligrams of vitamin C in his daily regimen. Since then, he states, he has not had a single cold. By investigation, the Nobel laureate was able to establish a complex series of reactions, too technical to reproduce here, between ascorbic acid and quinones produced by the splitting of the glucosides of wheat germ, the reactions being triggered by the manganese content of the wheat germ.

What it comes down to is that materials present in most plant foods to a very limited extent are present most richly in wheat germ. Thus, it is the belief of Dr. Szent-Györgyi that most any plant food we eat will add to the potency of vitamin C intake to some extent, increasing its beneficial effect. But to activate fully the large amounts of vitamin C recommended by him, by Linus Pauling and by growing numbers of other scientists, he believes that two ounces or more of wheat germ every day is a necessity. "My finding wheat germ useful against colds is not at variance with Pauling's statements," says Szent-Györgyi. "If one is deficient in two factors, administration of one of them may help to some extent, while full benefit may be derived only by taking the two in combination."

When the scientist speaks of "full benefit," he is, of course, talking about far more than merely preventing colds, important as that single activity may be. It has already been mentioned that he believes the length and continued good health and activity of his life are attributable to the combination, and that is certainly more than a matter of just staying free of colds.

As is demonstrated biochemically in *The Living State,* vitamin C, as well as being a reducing agent, functions as an antioxidant in relation to a wide variety of toxic materials that, if permitted to oxidize in our systems, initiate chain reactions that disrupt the normal orderly processes of life.

Vitamin C prevents the oxidation. What the wheat germ does is furnish the vitamin C with otherwise missing chemical elements that permit the vitamin actually to regenerate itself so that it is not used up the first time it functions as an antioxidant but is able to perform the same protective role many times over.

It begins to look as though, in trying to put into a nutshell a description of the function of vitamin C, we would have to say that its role is to maintain the stable functioning of our bodies against the disrupting influences of the hundreds or thousands of types of stress to which we are continually being subjected.

No wonder Dr. Szent-Györgyi declares in *The Living State:*

I always felt that not enough use was made of ascorbic acid. "If we lack ascorbic acid we develop scurvy. If we do not have scurvy, we have enough ascorbic acid." So the argument ran; the logic was impeccable. The flaw in this argument is that scurvy is not the first symptom of deficiency. It is a sign of the final collapse of the organism, a premortal syndrome, and there is a very wide gap between scurvy and a completely healthy condition. Good health is the state in which we feel best, work best, and have greatest resistance to disease. Nobody knows how far we are from such a state. This could be established only by extensive statistical studies which are not available. Solutions to this problem are full of pitfalls. If, owing to inadequate food, you contract a cold and die of pneumonia your diagnosis will be pneumonia, not malnutrition, and chances are that your doctor will have treated you only for pneumonia.

Is our body such a poor mechanism that it has to break down every so often with a cold or other ailment? Or do we abuse our body, and feed it so poorly that its breakdown is comparable to the breakdown of an unlubricated engine? I am often shocked at the eating habits of people. What I find difficult to understand as a biologist is not why people become ill, but how they manage to stay alive at all. Our body must be a very wonderful instrument to withstand all our insults.

It is good, then, to realize that the simple addition of two ounces a day of wheat germ to our diets can fully activate our vitamin C intake and do so much to eliminate the chronic deficiency of this all-important vitamin from which we all seem to suffer, no matter how much we consume, simply because the vitamin is used inefficiently unless we use it in combination with wheat germ.

9 Hepatitis and Paralysis R in Season

If you were to ask me to name, among all the foods a fat man enjoys, the one food I would rather eat than any other, my answer would have to be steamed clams. I love them. The very odor sets my nose quivering and my gastric juices flowing. What's more, in nutritional terms, clams are among the finest foods one can eat.

I haven't had a clam in the past four years. I don't dare. And I consider myself lucky that I never got a bad one in the years before I learned that clams, too, can be as polluted as the water they live in. The situation has been a serious one for better than ten years now.

In November, 1963, a Connecticut housewife was suddenly afflicted with an illness that seemed to strike her everywhere at once. She had swollen glands in her neck and armpits, she ran a fever, and her skin developed a yellowish tinge. There were pain and tenderness on the right side of her abdomen. She was tired and listless, depressed, had no appetite and suffered from chronic headaches. She waited five days for the trouble to go away before going to her doctor, who was not able to do much for her except to give her medicines that made her feel a little better during the months it took for her body to heal itself.

This woman had never eaten a clam in her life. But her husband had, and that was enough to give her infectious hepatitis.

The case was one of 448—an epidemic—that occurred in the state of Connecticut at that time as a result of the consumption of clams. The epidemic was described and reported in the article "An Epidemic of Clam-Associated Hepatitis" in the *Journal of the American Medical Association* (April 28, 1969). In it six public-health physicians, Dr. Shaun Ruddy, Dr. Donald Johnson, Dr. James Mosley, Dr. John Atwater, Dr. Michael Rossetti and Dr. James Hart, warn that the same kind of epidemic can recur at any time and that it is just about impossible for any of the present control methods actually to make certain that clams are clean.

During the Connecticut epidemic investigators found that in 123 of the 448 cases the victims ate raw clams themselves. How the rest were given the disease cannot be stated absolutely, but of course hepatitis is *infectious,* communicable by direct person-to-person contact.

In January, 1964, when it had become clear that an epidemic was under way, the public-health officials began investigating, looking for a way to trace the source and put an end to the rapid spread of the disease. And what is truly shocking is they found it impossible to do so. To demonstrate why the situation could not be medically controlled, they describe clam marketing practices in their AMA *Journal* article.

Harvesters are self-employed clammers dependent for their living on their ability to find clams in sea water, harvest and sell them. They are supposed to confine their harvesting to waters that have been approved for the purpose. But suppose they can make a bigger catch by going outside the prescribed limits? Who is going to know? The harvester sells his catch to a distributor, known as a primary shipper. The primary shipper sorts them not by source, but by size, packing the size-graded clams in bushel bags.

"An individual harvester's catch, if sold either to a small dealer or during a period of low sales volume, may be distributed among two or three bags. On the other hand, if sold to a larger dealer or at a busy time of year, any one catch may be represented by a few clams in many different bags, with potentially wide geographic distribution." Thus, by the time the clams leave the primary shipper, it is already impossible to pinpoint the source of any bad ones. And that is only the beginning.

The primary shipper in turn sells to a number of reshippers, who in turn sell to retail markets and restaurants. "At each level of marketing, purchasing from multiple sources is practiced in an attempt to assure a steady supply when shellfish are scarce. . . . Despite the requirement that a tag indicating the growing area and registration number of the primary shipper be affixed to each bag, resale by reshippers can easily result in inability to trace any given bushel bag. This difficulty is compounded by 'lending,' a practice in which primary shippers or reshippers exchange various quantities of clams among themselves."

In other words, an investigator may know that a case of viral hepatitis occurred after clams were eaten at a particular restaurant. He goes to the restaurant and finds that it bought its clams from three or four different reshippers, and there is no way of telling which one sold the bad clams. What is more, the reshippers really don't know the origin of the clams that they sold. So the governmental requirement of a tag to indicate the growing area is rendered absolutely meaningless, and when clams turn out to have come from polluted water, there is no way of discovering what water that is and banning further harvesting of clams there.

Furthermore, it takes from fifteen to forty-five days for the disease to incubate; in that time the virus-bearing clams can be spread far and wide. "There were 61 restaurants and 20 retail markets from which patients with hepatitis had purchased raw clams during the two months prior to the onset of the illness. Some of these establishments were supplied directly by primary shippers and others by one or more of 22 reshippers. No single restaurant, market, or reshipper could account for more than a few cases." Shipments of the same clams were spread out throughout the Northeast from Rhode Island to Pennsylvania.

All of the above explores only the possibility of getting bad clams from "legal" fishing waters that have become contaminated since their last inspection. The AMA *Journal* article, however, points out that illegal harvesting from waters known to be polluted, called bootlegging, also occurs despite the best law-enforcement efforts.

There is only one sane conclusion. The best efforts of government are inadequate and there is no way of truly policing the harvesting of shellfish—particularly clams—so that the consumer can be sure they will not sicken him. "That the responsible shellfish may well have come from open waters is suggested by the continued distribution of contaminated clams through regular channels at a time when intensive policing was in effect. Open areas are periodically sampled for bacteriological quality. Such sampling, however, may fail to detect intermittent contamination. In addition, bacterial counts may be an inadequate index of viral contamination." And the authors conclude that as pollution of our coastal waters increases it is going to become even more difficult to be sure that shellfish are safe to eat.

What kind of pollution is involved?

It is simply raw or insufficiently treated sewage dumped into the ocean by thousands of municipalities. Shellfish live and breed in waters close to shore, and so they are particularly vulnerable to contamination. The commonest, though far from the only ill result, is hepatitis.

It is a commonly held belief that the hepatitis virus is present only in raw shellfish, like cherrystones and little necks on the half shell. Not so, say Dr. Raymond Koff, Dr. George Grady, Dr. Thomas Chalmers and Dr. James Mosley who have made an intensive study of the situation. Their report "Importance of Exposure to Shellfish in a Nonepidemic Period" was issued in the *New*

England Journal of Medicine March 30, 1967. "Most steamer lovers cook the clams only until they open. This," according to Dr. Raymond S. Koff of Harvard Medical School, "leaves them almost raw—which is exactly the way steam clam lovers want them."

He pointed out that clams usually will open in a few minutes of steaming at 158 degrees F., whereas at least five minutes or more of steaming at 212 degrees F. is needed to kill the hepatitis virus. Such steaming, however, destroys the texture and flavor, so why bother?

Before the doctors made their study, it was widely believed that clams and oysters were only occasionally contaminated and could transmit hepatitis to man only intermittently when there was a shellfish-caused epidemic, five of which have occurred in the United States over the past eleven years. But clams and oysters present a *continual* hepatitis threat, says Dr. Koff, who carried out his study in ten Boston hospitals with Dr. George F. Grady and Dr. Thomas C. Chalmers of Tufts Medical School and Dr. James W. Mosley, chief of the Hepatitis Surveillance Unit of the United States Public Health Service, Atlanta.

The doctors also deflated another myth. At one time it was considered safe to consume shellfish in those months which had an *r* in their names. This survey revealed that disease from shellfish is now a threat twelve months of the year.

While person-to-person contact has generally been believed to be the most common cause of the spread of infectious hepatitis, when Koff studied 270 adult patients in the Boston area between 1963 and 1966, when the incidence of hepatitis was declining, he concluded that the ingestion of raw shellfish and steamed clams was as common a source of infection as contact with jaundiced persons, at least during this period.

The doctors urged that sanitation inspections of shellfish be tightened so that "the consumer should have some warranty that the shellfish that he is eating uncooked or partially cooked came from safe waters." Unfortunately, despite the best efforts of our inspectors, there seems to be no such thing as safe waters any more. As much as 6 percent of the shellfish sampled at random in 1971 from so-called safe waters were contaminated with unsatisfactory levels of bacteria. Inspectors in New York, New Jersey and Delaware (where three-fourths of the nation's clams are harvested) are spread so thin they can't begin to do an adequate policing job. And, even if they could, they lack the power actually to seize any shellfish that they find contaminated. Even if they could seize them, by the time laboratory tests are run to assess the contamination, the shellfish have already reached the market and could be on your table. Such were the alarming findings of a recent Associated Press survey (March 24, 1971).

The study indicated that there are so few inspectors they cannot possibly do a proper job, and inspection schedules go unmet. New York, for example, has only three inspectors to police 4,400 firms which dig, process or ship shellfish. To complicate the problem of the inspectors, offshore dumping of chemicals, sewage sludge and other wastes is virtually unpoliced.

The state agencies, besides being undermanned, are further hamstrung by the lack of tough measures with which to deal with offenders. Thus, the first time a shipper is caught with shellfish exceeding the maximum fecal coliform bacteria count of 230 parts per million, he is merely told of the contamination. A gentle slap on the wrist, but the shellfish go to market. The second time, his control processes are reviewed, but his shellfish could still be in your favorite restaurant. The third time, he may be denied permission to ship shellfish between states. He can still ship them city to city within the borders of the state. In fact, officials could not recall a single incident where a shipper's registration was revoked.

Among the solutions suggested for the thorny problem is that of depuration—or making the shellfish pure again. It is done by putting oysters, clams and mussels from polluted water into purified water for a period of time—long enough to permit them to rid themselves of bacterial organisms from sewage. The shellfish are placed in large tanks capable of holding several thousand. In the tank is water sterilized by ultraviolet radiation and aerated by cascade. After such purification, the oysters are tested for *E. coli,* a contaminating organism that comes from human feces. When found to be pure, they are released for sale and human consumption.

It sounds great, but it doesn't necessarily work. Dr. G. O. Barrow and Dr. D. C. Miller of the Public Health Laboratory, Royal Cornwall Hospital in England, said in *Lancet* (August 23, 1969) in a paper titled "Marine Bacteria in Oysters Purified for Human Consumption" that there is a different kind of danger in these oysters. While the oysters were, indeed, free of coliform bacteria, they had meanwhile accumulated other marine bacteria which destroy red blood cells in the human body. The depuration process may knock off some bacteria while it strengthens others.

For instance, an outbreak of gastroenteritis associated with eating oysters was reported in the *British Medical Journal* (May 16, 1970). The guilty oysters had been considered safe. They had been purified before going to market. They were served at a small dinner party, and almost all the guests became deathly sick with diarrhea, nausea, vomiting, malaise, aches, pains and fever.

It was pointed out by Ebba Waerland of Seewis-Dorf, Switzerland, that the irradiation process itself is fraught with unseen danger (*Archives of Clinical Ecology,* 1969). "In contrast to sterilization by heat," Waerland warns, "the various types of microorganisms differ in their reaction to irradiation and the spores are in general considerably more resistant than living germs. Certain types of microflora may remain more or less active. Highly resistant biotypes may survive, or by mutation, renew their activity and lead to a new microflora. A very special danger lies in the fact that in the foodstuffs a certain irradiation-resistant type may remain after irradiation and build up toxins, even though others may be destroyed." Thus, depuration with ultraviolet radiation can create problems more serious than those it solves.

There is also the ever-present danger of paralytic poisoning from eating mussels, soft-shell clams, oysters, sand crabs, shrimps, crabs and lobsters. Earl McFarren of the Public Health Service, in an article "Paralytic Shellfish Poison" in the publication *Advances in Food Research* (Vol. 10, Academic Press, N.Y., 1960) reports that by 1953 there were more than four hundred cases of mussel and clam poisoning recorded in the medical literature, including thirty-five deaths. Authorities agree that this represents only a fraction of those that actually occur but are never diagnosed or reported to recording centers.

In the summer of 1968 the Northumbrian coast of Britain was hit with an epidemic of paralytic shellfish poisoning that sent eighty-five persons to the hospital. Because of the British habit of boiling mussels thoroughly in water which is then discarded, there were, happily, no fatalities in this epidemic.

Americans were not quite so fortunate in the big epidemic of shellfish poisoning that hit San Francisco in 1927, when six of the 102 people affected died.

The symptoms of shellfish poisoning are fast and frightening. The victim notices a slight tingling and numbness of the lips within five to thirty minutes, then loss of strength in his muscles. After four to six hours, he is able to raise his head or move his arms or legs only with great difficulty. The longest recorded interval between eating poisonous shellfish and death is twelve hours and the shortest is two hours.

Because the poison acts so swiftly, remember to act at once should you happen to encounter it. The usual practice is to induce vomiting with an emetic, or purge with a strong laxative. But doctors agree that these measures cannot always be relied upon to intercept a fatal dose of poison. As soon as difficult breathing develops, artificial respiration should be applied, sometimes for several hours. In severe cases, this procedure may save a life.

The source of the poison is a marine organism, a one-cell toxic plant which appears among plankton—tiny sea creatures—when the water warms, usually in the summertime. The shellfish eat the plankton and, at the same time, ingest this poisonous organism, which they concentrate in their livers. "The mollusks are apparently unharmed, but the heat-stable poison can be lethal for many," says Dr. Rodney R. Beard, Department of Preventive Medicine, Stanford University Medical Center in a letter to the *New England Journal of Medicine* (July 21, 1966).

Seafood which carries disease and poison has no telltale appearance, has no off-taste to warn you of danger. When you eat it, you may be taking your first step toward a hospital bed—and you may find some of your close associates following you there, whether they ate the shellfish with you or merely dropped by to say "Hi" and shake hands.

With conditions what they are, there is only one realistic way that you and I can protect ourselves against the threat of shellfish contamination. We have to give up that particular pleasure and stop eating shellfish. There is no prophylactic we can take, no inspection system that can give us anything like believable assurances of purity.

Shellfish, given the chance, will feed on human feces. And there is no way on this earth that we can know whether that fresh, succulent clam or oyster on the plate has had the chance.

10 Fish Is Still Good Food

Who will ever forget the swordfish and tuna-fish scare of 1970? On a suggestion by his wife and students, Professor Bruce McDuffie of the State University at Binghamton, New York, analyzed a can of tuna fish for mercury content as something of a joke. To his amazement, he found that the mercury in the tuna ran well over the one-half part per million that the Food and Drug Administration had set up as a permissible level of contamination.

Professor McDuffie reported his finding to New York State health authorities and then, perhaps because he didn't want to be ignored, to the press as well. There is a strong tendency on the part of public-health agencies to shut their eyes to unpleasant facts, which might cause public panic. But, with the press already in possession of the facts, there was nothing to be done but investigate further. The regional laboratory of the FDA checked it out further and had to admit that, despite supposed federal monitoring, some 23 percent of the cans of tuna fish tested had high mercury content. The discovery led to the embarrassed recall of 921,-600 cans of tuna.

The incident led Professor McDuffie to believe that other fish ought to be checked for their mercury content as well, and that perhaps the federal government could not be relied on to do it.

He and his students bought some specimens from markets and fish stores. They were able to give a clean bill of health to cod, flounder, haddock and halibut, but when they checked out a swordfish steak, they were utterly horrified. The swordfish, they found, contained even more mercury than tuna.

The FDA, even while recalling nearly a million cans of tuna and temporarily banning swordfish from the market, hastened to reassure the public that there was no reason to panic. When I read those reassurances, my heart sank. I've always been prone to suspect that the FDA places a higher value on public confidence than it does on public health and began quietly looking into where I could get emergency treatment for my daughter, who has always loved tuna fish. Almost as bad, until we could get to the bottom of the question of mercury pollution of the water, we felt we had to play it safe and give up smoked salmon for Sunday breakfasts and our occasional pickled herring snacks with a before-dinner cocktail. This right on top of our forced abandonment of steamed clams! I was beginning to wonder if life was even worth living.

Fortunately, the Food and Drug Administration, perhaps to its own surprise—and certainly to mine—turned out to be right. When a later investigation of the toxicity of mercury was made by H. E. Ganther and his associates of the Department of Nutritional Sciences of the University of Wisconsin, the truly surprising discovery was made that the more tuna fish there is in the diet the fewer toxic effects can be expected from mercury. Feeding to Japanese quail and to rats doses of mercury that would be considered lethal or close to it for people, the investigators found that they could kill from 50 percent to 100 percent of their experimental animals. But when the diet was altered to contain 17 percent tuna by weight, there was almost complete protection.

The reason for this effect will be explored later in this chapter. For now it is probably enough for all of us to breathe a deep sigh of relief as we understand that all those tuna-sandwich lunches, even if they did contain some mercury, may actually have been protecting us against mercury poisoning. And, if you want further quick confirmation of that, just consider that museum specimens of tuna now in the Smithsonian Institution in Washington, caught at various times ranging from sixty-three to ninety-four years ago, have been found to contain as much mercury as the fresh tuna being analyzed today. There are people like the fishermen of the Azores, whose chief meat throughout their lives has been tuna and who have therefore been eating the mercury that tuna accumulate from ocean water yet have never shown any sign of mercury poisoning.

Of course, this is not to say that mercury in fish has no dangers. For example, a New York woman who for a period of five or six years was in the habit of eating from twelve to fourteen ounces of swordfish a day, as the basis of a reducing diet, developed symptoms that probably resulted from mercury poisoning—shaking hands, blurred vision, dizziness, great sensitivity to light and loss of memory. An analysis of her hair showed a very high mercury content, and though it was never actually proven that the swordfish she ate was the only source of mercury, it still seems likely that her diet was actually the cause of her troubles. This appears to have been a rare case, though, and in the quantities in which people normally eat swordfish, say once a week or less, there is no real reason to believe it dangerous.

And still mercury is a dangerous poison, while the question of when it is or isn't poisonous is a fairly subtle one.

Dr. Leonard J. Goldwater, professor of Community Health Sciences at Duke University, who is considered an authority on mercury, stated in "Mercury in the Environment" in *Scientific American* (May, 1971) that, if you were to swallow a pound or more of the pure mercury used in thermometers, you would suffer no significant adverse effect. On the other hand, if you are a dentist who uses mercury to make amalgam fillings and don't protect yourself against breathing the vaporized mercury that rises from the amalgam, you might find yourself with a perpetual cough, a painful tightness of the chest resembling angina, and, in extreme cases, possible fatal destruction of lung tissue. Mercury vapor is a killer. Pure liquid mercury is also toxic, but not enough so to be greatly feared.

When we speak of mercury as a pollutant, however, we are talking about something else again. We are talking about methyl mercury, an organic compound that is foreign to the sea.

In Japan, between 1953 and 1960, 121 people contracted what became known as Minamata disease. All lived on the periphery of Minamata Bay. Their symptoms included progressive blindness, loss of hearing, failure of coordination, tremors and deterioration of the mind. Forty-six of them died. There is no doubt that Minamata disease was caused by the eating of mercury-contaminated fish from Minamata Bay. They were poisoned by methyl mercury, an organic form of the metal, that was being discharged into the water from plastic manufacturing plants.

In the winter of 1970 it was found that seven members of a family named Huckleby in Alamogordo, New Mexico, had been poisoned by eating pork from a hog that had been fed seed grain that had been treated with a fungicide containing methyl mercury. Three of the children suffered severe brain damage.

Methyl mercury and other less common organic forms are highly poisonous in minute quantities. As well as occurring as industrial waste, they are formed on the bottoms of rivers, lakes and canals when inorganic mercury is put into the water and sinks. Mercury has a chemical affinity for certain special forms of protein, the sulfur-containing amino acids, and because of that affinity it becomes attached to microscopic organisms living in the sediment of fresh water. Unfortunately for us, the bacteria convert the mercury into methyl mercury, in which form it is more soluble and is diffused into the water. From the water it is concentrated in the bodies of fish.

If we eat fish contaminated with methyl mercury, we will be poisoned.

And, as the waste of eighty or ninety industrial processes, mercury is being dumped into water, where it becomes methylated. Paint manufacture, paper making, plastics, metal refining, drug manufacture and a host of others all use mercury—and for the most part dump the waste into the nearest body of water. Often the dumped waste is already in the poisonous methylated form.

It is only fish from the inland waters where mercury is dumped that can give us mercury poisoning, in the informed opinion of Dr. Henry Schroeder, director of the Trace Elements Laboratory of the Dartmouth Medical School. He would not advise anybody, for instance, to eat fish from Lake St. Clair, a beautiful lake near Detroit and Sarnia, Ontario, that has had so much mercury dumped into it that it has probably become permanently polluted.

Some of the more important inland waters that have been labeled mercury polluted by the Sierra Club are Lake Erie; the Mississippi River in Louisiana and Tennessee; the Delaware River in Delaware; the Androscoggin and Penobscot rivers in Maine; the Columbia River in Washington; the Ohio River in West Virginia.

It is well worth the trouble to avoid fish from these waters and others that you think might be mercury polluted. If in doubt, and if it's a fresh-water fish, don't eat it. Methyl-mercury poisoning can be treated medically. You swallow drugs that have a chemical affinity for the metal and little by little carry it out of the system. But it takes months to get rid of it all. And meanwhile, if poisoned, you will experience some remarkably unhappy symptoms and risk permanent brain damage.

So if there's any question in your mind about the origin of that whitefish, pike or trout, you'd better stick to ocean fish such as flounder, bluefish, halibut, and especially herring and tuna.

Why especially?

Because those fish tend to accumulate from sea water a mineral named selenium. And selenium is the only thing yet discovered that can protect us against the toxic effects of mercury. That effect was discovered in Czechoslovakia at the Institute of Physiology in Prague by J. Parizek and associates some seven or eight years ago. Using selenium compounds (pure selenium is all but nonexistent) administered to test animals prior to dosing them with mercury compounds of known poisonous nature, the Czech scientists found that it took only traces of selenium or other selenium compounds to afford complete protection against the toxic effects of the mercury. The studies of Parizek and his co-workers, which were extensive and thorough, suggested that the selenium somehow reacts with mercury within the body, rendering it harmless.

The study was generally forgotten until the tuna scare of 1970. After that, a team of investigators from the Department of Nutritional Sciences of the University of Wisconsin, led by H. E. Ganther, obtained some two thousand pounds of canned tuna that contained mercury in excess of the content permitted by the FDA. After analysis to confirm that the fish did indeed contain from .7 to 1 part per million of mercury, it was sprayed with methyl mercury hydroxide to build up the poisonous content and fed to Japanese quail, who were also fed a variety of experimental diets, varying quantities of the tuna being combined with a corn-soya mash which had also been liberally sprayed with methyl mercury hydroxide.

To the surprise of the investigators, they found that, in spite of the lethal quantities of methyl mercury, it was very hard to kill the quail if their diets also contained a good amount of the supposedly inedible tuna. Even though the amounts of methyl mercury received were identical, only 7 percent of the quail with tuna in their feed died, in contrast to 52 percent of those without it. (If you think that 7 percent isn't a terribly comforting figure, remember that the amount of methyl mercury in the quails' diet was astronomical compared to anything you might come across.)

Ganther and his associates believed that the fact that tuna *always* accumulate more selenium than mercury in their flesh is the determining factor that made the supposedly dangerous tuna actually a protector against methyl mercury. To check that conclusion they fed rats drinking water containing various concentrations of methyl mercury while their solid food either did or did not contain one-half part per million of selenium. Ten parts per million of methyl mercury failed to kill the rats getting the selenium.

The evidence seems fairly conclusive. Selenium is what protects us from methyl mercury. And the really strange thing about that is that selenium, if we get too much of it, is also poisonous. It is too much selenium in pasture grass that gives cattle the blind staggers. So there is no point in rushing out to get a selenium supplement for yourself. I don't believe it is even included in any general mineral supplement—and properly not. It would be far too easy to take too much of it.

There is virtually no chance, however, of receiving a toxic amount of selenium from food, while it is easy to make sure that you get enough to protect you from any methyl mercury you might inadvertently swallow. You simply make sure that your diet frequently contains foods with a high selenium content. Tuna is one of the leaders. Pickled herring—or any form of herring—is fine. Broccoli, onions, cabbage, asparagus, mushrooms and tomatoes all contain selenium. And, if you happen to be on a health-food kick and take brewer's yeast and wheat germ, you have it made. Aside from protection against organic mercury compounds, there is reason to believe that regular minute traces of selenium in the diet may protect against some forms of cancer and have an age-retarding effect as well. So you really can't go wrong with it. Nevertheless, I'd still stay away from fresh-water fish unless you're absolutely sure where it was caught. But ocean fish are fine, and in the case of some, are actually protection against mercury. Enjoy.

The dangers of eating fish are few and far between. If you choose from those varieties that are safe and wholesome, you probably should be eating more fish. There is good reason to believe that you can improve your general health and more particularly your heart health by simply replacing other protein foods with fish a few times a week. Physicians at the University of California recently conducted studies which involved close to four hundred men who were placed on a diet which included three to five seafood meals a week over a period of two to three years. The results were lowered cholesterol counts, a loss of excess weight and a general feeling of well-being. In the booklet *Reduce Your Risk of Heart Attack,* the American Heart Association suggests that a high-seafood diet would be good for anybody.

Most nutritionists believe that fish is one of the finest foods anyone can eat. Few foods have more of what it takes to maintain a healthy circulatory system than seafood. Fish is low in calories; it has almost no weight-producing carbohydrates or saturated fats. Its rich supply of unsaturated oils actually helps dissolve any cholesterol accumulations in the bloodstream. Fish protein is the best there is, and because protein foods are metabolized more slowly than starchy ones, it satisfies the appetites of overeaters without the accompanying dangers of too much food. Fresh, untreated fish is practically free of sodium, a common restriction for heart patients. If doctors were commissioned to invent the ideal food for a heart patient, chances are they would come up with fish, or something close to it.

Fish is also a relatively inexpensive protein source. The protein in any fish is at least as good as that of meat, but fish is often cheaper. Fish protein is complete; that is, it supplies the full range of protein elements (amino acids) we need for good health. Compare the amino acids of chicken and beef with those of fish and you will find that fish has at least as much to offer as either of them.

When you get your protein from fish, 97 percent of it will be absorbed by your system and that is 10 percent more than your system can utilize from any other source except egg or milk.

Fish is high in iron, iron that is rapidly absorbed. To the heart patient, iron means more-efficient blood composition, and this in turn means less work for the heart. The thyroid gland needs iodine (and fish has plenty) to produce the thyroxine that works toward proper growth, proper use of carbohydrates, quick reactions and normal heart action. These mineral contents of fish are particularly important to women. Most women, because of monthly blood loss, tend to need more dietary iron than men. Many women, and particularly teenage girls, are anemic or on the borderline of becoming so. And iodine, for rather complicated metabolic reasons, helps to keep a woman from developing breast cancer. Women can better their chances of avoiding both problems simply by incorporating enough fish in their diets.

Though the B vitamins have made their reputation as protectors of the nervous system, their effect on the circulation and health of the heart is extremely important. According to the classic text *Avitaminosis,* by Walter Eddy, Ph.D., and Gilbert Dalldorf, M.D. (Williams and Wilkins, Baltimore, 1944), "B-vitamin deficiency impairs the function of the heart, increases the tendency to extravascular fluid collections and results in terminal cardiac standstill." Dr. James S. McLester tells of experiments with pigs that were fed diets deficient in thiamine (B_1) and showed scarring of the right side of the heart. (*Nutrition and Diet in Health and Disease,* W. B. Saunders Company, 1949.)

Classic symptoms of beriberi, a disease of vitamin-B deficiency, are heart damage, decreased circulation time, and a rise in blood pressure. The effect of thiamine on the heart and circulatory system is to increase arterial tone, according to Dr. Eddy and Dr. Dalldorf. In the face of this information it is comforting to know that the B complex is about as high in fish as in any food, except perhaps liver.

Of course the beneficial action of these nutrients is not tied exclusively to improving or preserving the health of the heart. The proteins, vitamins and minerals of fresh fish offer remarkable dividends in the health of the nerves, bones, skin and other organs. They also protect the body against invading infections and degenerative disorders.

Commercial fertilizers and insecticides play no part in the fish business, and while the pollution of inland waters does contaminate most fresh-water fish, ocean fish are still free of all but negligible traces of agricultural chemicals. Preservatives, artificial flavorings and colorings cannot be used on fish. Ocean fish are not doped, treated with chemicals, or processed. Fish taken from the great fishing banks far out to sea come to us unpolluted and in so many varieties you would be wise indeed to serve fish more frequently and avoid in some measure the hormones and antibiotics which contaminate most of this nation's meat.

The vitamin content of fish, though always high, is subject to seasonal change. The content of vitamin A is highest in summer, but also remains very high in the winter months, as compared with other foodstuffs, for example butter. The flesh of fatty fish or dark-meat fish is higher in these vitamins than is that of the white-fleshed fish.

Strange though it may seem, fish is low in sodium. This goes for ocean fish as well as fresh-water fish and is one reason why fish is so frequently prescribed for patients with high blood pressure. It is also high in phosphorus, which is necessary to the brain and is probably where fish got its reputation as a brain food. Calcium, too, is found in fish in a form which is just as absorbable as that found in milk. But the very important and scarce mineral magnesium is higher in fish than it is in milk.

Taken all in all, you couldn't find a better food. I find it heartening that in spite of the heedless pollution of the earth's waters, so much fish remains clean and wholesome.

11 Survival in a Radioactive World

Leukemia kills about 2,100 American children a year, more than died of polio in 1952, the peak year for that disease, according to *Health Topics* (October, 1970) published by the *Congressional Quarterly*. How much of this heartbreaking suffering is the result of radioactive fallout, the devastating aftermath of nuclear testing?

According to one radiation health expert, Professor E. J. Sternglass of the department of radiology of the University of Pittsburgh, the incidence of childhood leukemia doubled in the Albany-Troy, New York, area over an eight-year period as a result of radioactive fallout dumped there during a 1953 rainstorm after a nuclear-weapons test in Nevada. He told a meeting of the Health Physics Society in June, 1968, that there were twenty cases of leukemia in the one-to-ten age group during the eight years before the fallout and forty-two cases in the same age group during the eight years following. The tragic consequences, according to Professor Sternglass, affected children in their mothers' wombs and children born as long as ten years after the incident.

We haven't seen much in the newspapers lately about strontium 90 and many of us have forgotten that only a few years ago the very thought of what horrible mischief this dangerous element could perpetrate on us, and on future generations, struck terror to the very marrow of our radioactive bones.

Aside from the obvious fact that in the area of a nuclear explosion intense radiation poisoning can lead to death within a week, in lesser degrees exposure has brought an increased incidence of leukemia, bone cancer and a wide range of illness and symptoms from stillbirths to deformed babies to spontaneous abortions and sterility.

Has the absence of information on the strontium 90 in the atmosphere lulled us into a false sense of security? True, aboveground and atmospheric testing of nuclear weapons has dwindled, with only France and China still conducting aboveground tests, but this does not mean there is no more radioactivity in our environment. Some portion of the radioactive poison that nuclear weapons have added to our environment will endure practically forever. The load diminishes slightly with time, but as Surgeon General Dr. Luther L. Terry and PHS Radiology Chief Dr. Donald R. Chadwick pointed out in the AMA *Journal* (June 23, 1962), "There is no level of radiation exposure below which there can be absolute certainty that harmful effects will not occur to at least a few individuals when sufficiently large numbers of people are exposed."

That is why more and more scientists are exploring ways in which we may all help our systems to eliminate radioactive matter. For the simple fact is that, while nuclear-weapon production is slowing down, atomic power plants are proliferating. And, as shown by Professor Sternglass in his new book *Low-Level Radiation* (Pyramid Books, New York, 1973) each nuclear power plant and to a much greater extent each nuclear-fuel processing plant releases radiation into the atmosphere. Furthermore, as each plant gets older, the amount of radioactive gases released increases sharply. The result, Professor Sternglass demonstrates convincingly, has been an increase in the number of infants dying of respiratory failure and children dying of leukemia and a spectacular rise in adults "suffering from all types of chronic lung disease around the world, multiplying the effects of other pollutants—including cigarettes."

Until now, according to Dr. Sternglass's information, most of the human damage from atomic power plants has been confined to the immediate vicinity of those plants. What will happen, however, if all the electric power companies are permitted to proceed unchecked with their plans for new nuclear power plants? Almost every power company in the United States has such plans. What is going to happen if we get so many nuclear power plants that, no matter where you live, you still find yourself near one? If Professor Sternglass and other authorities are to be believed, there is going to be a vast increase in infant mortality, a far greater incidence of leukemia, far more of a type of anemia characterized by destruction of the blood platelets, and far greater incidence of emphysema and lung cancer.

No less prestigious a group than the National Academy of Sciences' National Research Council released a report in November, 1972, which said that the present Atomic Energy Commission guideline for human exposure to radiation is far higher than it should be. The scientists who participated in the report estimated that Americans on the average receive about 100 milli-rems a year from natural background sources such as cosmic rays, radioactive material in rocks and other sources. In addition, the medical uses of radiation subject every American to an average dose of roughly an additional 100 milli-rems. The scientists calculated that an average dose of 170 milli-rems for the general population could cause 100 to 1,800 cases of serious genetic diseases in the first year. The numbers would increase as the number of radiation-caused genetic mutations accumulated in the overall population.

According to the report, the present increment of radiation from the nuclear power industry is about one milli-rem a year, or about one percent of the natural background. Although the figure seems small, most of the scientists who oppose nuclear power plants do so because too little is known about the future effects of increasing the background radiation by even a small amount. Keep building new nuclear plants, multiply their number by 10 or 20, and the increment will become 20 or 30 milli-rems. That's every year, so that ten years from now we could easily find the background radiation has increased to 130 milli-rems—a frighteningly dangerous level.

"It is true that all living things have adapted themselves to natural radiation," wrote Sir Ritchie Calder in *Living with the Atom* (University of Chicago Press, 1962). "But what can happen to a species through eons of time is something different from rashly increasing artificial radiation in the course of a few years, with our imperfect knowledge of the harm that may be done." In other words, we just don't know what the long-term effects of increased radiation are. But, if the scheduled nuclear plants are built (one thousand are planned to be in operation by the year 2000), adding numerous milli-rems to the earth's surface, future generations will find out.

There are some things that we do know, however, and they provide enough food for thought.

In the town of Aliquippa, Pennsylvania, nine miles away from the Shippingport Nuclear Generating Plant, the mortality rate for infants is more than double that for the rest of the state. There is more than twice as much leukemia as the state average and infant diseases of all kinds amount to 165 percent of the state average. Leukemia and infant mortality have been declining throughout Pennsylvania—but not in Aliquippa. The figures were uncovered by Dr. Sternglass when he was asked by the owner of the plant, Duquesne Light Co., to make such a survey.

Naturally, when the facts emerged, Duquesne Light attacked them. But the only defense it could muster was a claim that the black population of Aliquippa has increased, weighting the health statistics. A quick check of U.S. Census figures showed that the black population has actually decreased. A further claim that the high rate of sickness and death are due to nonradioactive air pollution was not taken seriously, since that type of pollution is the same in Aliquippa as everywhere else in western Pennsylvania.

Duquesne Light, in self-defense, contracted for another study by National Utilities Service Corp. The study was assigned for analysis to Professor Morris DeGroot, head of the Department of Statistics at Carnegie-Mellon University.

DeGroot's studies confirmed Sternglass's.

It was shown that in 1970, the year of highest infant mortality in Aliquippa, the level of strontium 90 in milk at the six local dairies also reached an all-time high. It was actually 75 percent higher than the average concentration for the region. Unwilling to believe their results, the National Utilities Service technicians repeated their measurements three times. After that there was no longer any room for doubt.

Thus, even from what is considered one of the safest of atomic power plants, there is a discharge of radioactive gases. Kept within the limits that the Atomic Energy Commission considers permissible, as the discharges are at Shippingport, the gases do contain radioactive strontium which falls to the ground. Because of its chemical affinity for calcium, the radioactive strontium gets into the grass and other high-calcium cattle feed. Through the feed it gets into the milk, and from the milk into the children.

It should also be remembered that while small children are the first to show the effects of fallout, and probably accumulate more because they are heavy milk drinkers, the effects are by no means limited to them. Radioactive minerals will be found in all food and adults accumulate them, too. Deposited into bone, they can cause bone cancer. They can damage chromosomes and result in defective or dead babies. And there is some reason to believe they can also simply shorten life, by affecting the nucleic acids, without causing any specific disease at all.

Yet not everybody will succumb to what the Atomic Energy

Commission likes to call "negligible" amounts of radioactive matter added to the atmosphere. The difference between those who become ill and those who stay healthy, those who die before their time and those who live out their natural lives, may well lie in their diets. And there is every reason to believe that a couple of simple, perfectly natural and palatable additions to our diets will spell this difference.

At the Gastrointestinal Research Laboratories of McGill University in Montreal it was discovered that giant brown kelp, a common seaweed that grows abundantly in the Pacific Ocean off the coast of California, contains sodium alginate, which can reduce by 50 to 80 percent the amount of radioactive strontium—strontium 90—absorbed through the intestine. Such a reduction is no small matter. It is true, of course, that if there are radioactive particles in the air some of them will be breathed in directly, and there is nothing kelp can do to prevent that. But the greatest absorption of fallout comes through the food we eat and the water we drink. It is particularly where calcium is to be found, in leafy green vegetables, in milk, in hard water, that strontium 90 tends to accumulate. It is the same affinity for calcium that makes strontium 90 the most dangerous of radioactive materials within the body. It goes straight for the bones, destroying the function of the bone marrow. Furthermore, strontium 90 is so similar in chemical structure to calcium that the body is unable to distinguish one from the other and in no way resists absorption of the pollutant. Sodium alginate, however, can make this distinction. According to Dr. Stanley Skoryna, one of the McGill University team that made the crucial study, sodium alginate "permits calcium to be absorbed through the intestinal walls, while it binds most of the strontium within the intestine." He described the process to the Seventh Annual International Congress of Gastro-enterology in Brussels in 1966. And what his description amounted to was that the sodium alginate in kelp, described as "a naturally-occurring, non-toxic, aciditic polysaccharide," can discriminate so successfully that it actually separates radioactive strontium from the calcium to which it is attached, binding the strontium in the intestine while permitting the calcium to be freely absorbed. The sodium alginate and the bound strontium are subsequently excreted, removing the radioactive material from the system.

In the Canadian study rats were both injected with strontium 89 and fed it in their drinking water. Strontium 89 is virtually identical to strontium 90 but has a much shorter half-life, making it a great deal safer to work with. They both have the same chemical reactions, and we can be sure that anything that removes strontium 89 from the system will do the same to strontium 90. After receiving the strontium 89 both by mouth and injection, some of the rats were also fed sodium alginate added to their feed. The animals protected with the kelp material showed 60 percent less strontium in their blood and 75 percent less in their bones than the control group.

There are some interesting numbers in the McGill University study, indicating that you don't really need a great deal of sodium alginate to protect you from the fallout you're going to receive from your friendly neighborhood nuclear power station. First, the rats in the study were challenged with fallout comparable to that of a nuclear bomb explosion. They were fed one-half micro-curie of strontium 89 for each gram of food. That means a test rat ate more radioactive material in a single day than we are ever likely to eat ourselves, barring nuclear war or an out-and-out explosion at the power station. And it took approximately three-and-a-half grams of sodium alginate to remove two-thirds of the strontium from their bodies. That is less than a tenth of an ounce.

The researchers could not determine whether more sodium alginate would do the job even better, because the experiment was limited by the appetites of small white rats that were certainly thrown off their feed by the strontium 89 they were given.

There is little doubt in my mind that just a few grams of sodium alginate—less than a quarter of an ounce—would do a superb and

very important job in protecting a person against radioactive strontium in the diet. It is especially important for milk-drinking children.

So where do you get sodium alginate, and what do you do
with it?

Sodium alginate is a common commercial product used indus-
trially as a thickener and stabilizer. Many brands of ice cream
contain it. Commercial bakeries use it in cake icings. As far as I
know, it might even be in sour cream and cottage cheese. But how
are we going to know? Food labels are uninformative and, as required by 1973 regulations of the Food and Drug Administration,
will soon be telling us nothing at all about what we're really eating. So there is no way to tell, and the only remedy is to add
sodium alginate to your own food at home. It has recently (fall,
1973) become available in health-food stores in one-pound containers and is also obtainable from mail order sellers of special
food products.

Once you have obtained it, you have to use a little imagination.
It's perfectly pleasant to use, and it is an effective transparent
thickening agent. So make your own gelatin desserts and aspics,
adding some sodium alginate. Putting up preserves? Sodium alginate helps. You can thicken soups and gravies with it. Or you can
figure out your own ways, including homemade ice cream. Use a
blender to add it to any liquid, otherwise it may clump.

It's surely worth a little trouble to add this protector to your
food and make sure that your children, at least, get a couple of
grams every day.

This process by which one material attaches to another and
bonds it firmly is known as chelation. It is a widely used medical
technique for removing undesirable materials from the body. The
trick is to find a substance that is itself inert within the human
digestive system—that will neither be altered by the digestive enzymes nor absorbed into the body—but that, in passing through

the digestive tract, will chelate the undesirable material, so that both will be excreted together.

There are materials that might be considered professional chelating agents, widely used by doctors. Some of them are resins similar to the resins used in water softeners. Some are pharmaceutical chemicals cleverly designed with an affinity for a wide range of metals. They are effective but have one drawback—all of them are at least somewhat toxic and the results of long-term use are largely unknown. Consequently, you can use them only under medical supervision and then not for a very long time. So, while sodium alginate is no more effective at removing radioactive strontium than other, previously known chelating agents, it is still superior and an important discovery, for fairly obvious reasons: it is a food material that is not known to have any toxic effects; because it is not known to have any toxic effects, it can be used freely without any help from a doctor; it is readily available and much cheaper than any equivalent pharmaceutical product, yet it is as effective as any other known chelating agent.

You will have gathered by now that I'm really enthusiastic about sodium alginate. Yet it is not the only nontoxic food material with that kind of protective quality. And on the premise that no chelate is necessarily 100 percent effective, it is surely worthwhile to know about the others.

The most obvious mineral to bind radioactive strontium is calcium. Actually, it is the strong affinity of the two minerals that makes the strontium isotope such a danger. Yet the very same quality that makes calcium an efficient medium for carrying radioactive strontium into the system makes it equally efficient at transporting the deadly material out again—if there is enough calcium to do it. Surplus calcium is either not absorbed and excreted fecally, carrying along with it any strontium it meets in the gut, or, if it does get into the bloodstream, is filtered out through the kidneys into the urine, again carrying strontium out of the system.

This effect was checked by Dr. H. Spencer, Dr. I. Lewin and Dr. J. Samachson of the Metabolic Section of the Veterans Administration Hospital, Hines, Illinois. In the *International Journal of Applied Radiation and Isotopes* (18: 407–415, 1967) they reported that they had administered both calcium and magnesium intravenously to hospital patients to study their effect on the radioactive strontium the patients were consuming in their diets. Injecting the minerals into the veins, of course, was a good way to make sure that they got into the bloodstream. It was found that each mineral, both separately and together, significantly increased the amount of radioactive strontium that was removed from the bloodstream and subsequently excreted. Tested in various ways, the same effect has been reported in a host of scientific journals ranging from the *New York State Journal of Medicine* to the highly technical *Health Physics.*

Magnesium, a mineral not previously discussed, is also as effective as calcium in carrying radioactive matter out of the body when the mineral itself is excreted. The reason it has not been mentioned up to now is that, unlike calcium, magnesium in the diet does not bring radioactive matter into the system because magnesium-rich foods tend to be well protected against contamination by strontium 89 and 90. The commonest high-magnesium foods are nuts and seeds of all kinds, which absorb into their shells any fallout that lodges on them but do not permit it to pass into the inner kernel that is actually eaten. Shellfish are also extremely high in magnesium content, but both the water in which they live and their own shells protect them from fallout contamination. So dietary magnesium, unlike high-calcium foods, represents pretty good protection against fallout without burdening the system by first carrying the strontium in. It must be remembered, however, that it is only the excess of either mineral that will be excreted and thus have this protective effect.

One good way of making sure you have such a surplus is to take a daily supplement of a readily available natural material known as dolomite. Dolomite is actually a common type of limestone which is about 40 percent magnesium carbonate. It occurs in mountainous formations, the upper surface of which is a natural trap for radioactive fallout. The stone that is mined from beneath is free of fallout. For dietary purposes the stone is pulverized, sterilized and then made into either a tablet or a powder.

It may seem strange to eat stone, but this particular stone is actually perfectly digestible and beneficial to the body. Besides, all the minerals in our food come from the earth or from stones. In fact, one leading antacid tablet that we take without a second thought has nearly the same mineral composition as dolomitic limestone. It is composed of calcium carbonate, magnesium carbonate and magnesium trisilicate. Dolomite is calcium carbonate and magnesium carbonate. So even though you would not normally pick up a chunk of stone and gnaw on it, the minerals the body obtains from dolomite are not only valuable for removing fallout—they are essential to health and to life itself. Without them, in fact, the heart would not beat.

In *Heart Journal* (March, 1967) Dr. Winifred Nayler of the Baker Medical Research Institute, Melbourne, Australia, describes the electrochemical process that takes place in each cell of the heart. On the outer surface of each heart-tissue cell, there is a thin filament known as actin. The actin reaches with a kind of magnetic attraction toward the center of the cell, shortening the cell's length. When many cells shorten at the same time, a muscle contracts. And it is calcium, fed to the actin by the bloodstream, that provides both the stimulus and the means by which the actin does its work. A shortage of calcium must inevitably result in a weakened heartbeat.

Still, Dr. Nayler tells us, while calcium is fundamentally necessary to the heartbeat, the calcium will not do what it is supposed to do unless it in turn is controlled by a sufficient quantity of magnesium in the system. The reason for this is that the actin must alternately absorb and release calcium. If it could not do both, the heart would either contract and stay contracted or else refuse to contract at all. For the heart to keep alternately contracting and relaxing requires that it be a very busy living chemical laboratory. And magnesium seems to be the key element that actually regulates heartbeat. How does it do this? By providing the tiny positive electrical charge that repels calcium, pushing it to the opposite side of the individual cell and reversing the contraction that has just taken place. Throughout the body, magnesium seems to be the mineral of basic importance in controlling the manner in which electrical charges are used to induce the passage of materials in and out of cells.

Nor is the heart the only part of the circulatory system that is affected and, in this way, controlled by whether we have enough magnesium in our diets. Throughout our systems, all the muscular tissues are designed to contract and relax, and if either function fails, there is trouble. Hypertension, or high blood pressure, is caused by an excessive contraction or reduced relaxation of the muscles surrounding the walls of arteries. It was reported in the *Journal of the American Medical Association* (February 22, 1965) by Dr. R. H. Seller that magnesium salts induced these muscles to relax and had therefore been found effective as a treatment for high blood pressure.

Similarly, in experimenting on cellular metabolism with possible treatments for arteriosclerosis (hardening of the arteries), Dr. T. Shimamoto reported in the *American Heart Journal* in 1969 that he was able to reduce swelling and consequent constriction of arterial walls with magnesium salts. According to Dr. Mildred Seelig (*American Journal of Clinical Nutrition,* June, 1964), there is a direct relationship between the amount of magnesium in the diet and ability to avoid high blood pressure. Dr. Seelig regards the difference in magnesium consumption as an important reason why there are far fewer heart attacks among Orientals than there are in the Western countries.

As research in biochemistry advances, scientists have come to realize how important is the long-known fact that our bodies are constantly generating and discharging tiny electrical impulses. These minute electrical charges were long regarded as a curiosity of no great significance, but it has been discovered that they are an essential part of the life processes. Every movement, external or internal, is triggered by such impulses transmitted along nerves. Without our electrical systems, there could be no life whatsoever. And so today we are compelled to recognize that, if magnesium is the primary regulator of the electrical activity in our bodies, then magnesium is obviously of far greater importance to health and life itself than anybody guessed even ten years ago. This being so, what chance is there that you are getting enough magnesium in your regular diet?

Dr. Seelig calculated that the average American falls short by 200 milligrams or more a day of the optimal amount of magnesium one should consume for good health. Present in many foods, magnesium is unfortunately extremely sensitive to heat and easily lost during processing. People who eat raw or unprocessed foods probably get enough. How many Americans do? How many Americans even find it possible?

If you assume that your own diet is average, with a daily 200-milligram deficit of magnesium, then you would need a supplementary intake of about 400 milligrams to secure an excretable surplus that would help you rid your body of radioactive strontium. A gram a day of dolomite will give you the 400 milligrams of magnesium and 600 milligrams of uncontaminated calcium. It can only do you good.

12 Lead—the Sweet Poison

A major controversy of the past few years, and one that is still raging, concerns the treatment of so-called hyperkinetic children— children who find it very hard to sit still, are easily excited, have a short attention span, and tend to ignore the rules and do as they please. They don't learn much in a classroom, and they are certainly a disruptive influence.

The number of hyperkinetic children is increasing every year, a phenomenon which will be explained in this section. But, for the moment, let's not quarrel with the standard psychiatric evaluation that these children suffer from "minimal brain damage." That means that medical diagnostic techniques don't show any damage, their intelligence is not retarded, their health seems all right and their family backgrounds are not particularly unusual. So, since the psychiatrists can't figure out why the children behave that way, they assume that their brains must be just a little damaged.

The solution? Drug the children into passivity. This technique was quietly but rapidly spreading through the nation's educational system when the scandal broke in Omaha.

In December, 1968, Dr. Byron R. Oberst, an Omaha pediatrician, attended a seminar at Syracuse University where he was sold on the value of using "behavior modification" drugs to treat "hyperactive" school children. He returned to Omaha, as he himself describes it, with a "new mission": to spread the word to his fellow physicians and to Omaha's school personnel.

A high-powered campaign to promote the drugging of children speedily got under way, once the drug-oriented physicians of the medical society got the message from their colleagues. The fact that the drugs carry grave dangers from side effects and that some are addictive was no deterrent. Seminars, a propaganda film called *Why Billy Can't Learn,* and a new organization, STAAR (Skills, Technique, Academic Accomplishment, and Remediation), all combined to show parents and teachers that a "difficult" or "hyperactive" child will improve ("be happier" and "learn better") if he's properly drugged.

It didn't take long for teachers to start spotting pupils who would "benefit" from drug therapy. Parents were persuaded—sometimes harassed—into getting drug treatment prescribed by family physicians or city clinics. By 1970 there were between three thousand and six thousand legally drugged pupils, from six-year-olds up, in Omaha's classrooms. As one Omaha educator commented in reference to the application of drugs to the problems of behavior: "I would say it's a growing field." The wave of the future!

The drugs used to quiet children in the Omaha experiment are, paradoxically, stimulants when taken by adolescents and adults. They include amphetamines like Dexedrine and a relatively new drug, Ritalin, unrelated to the amphetamines but also a stimulant with a quieting effect on "hyperactive" children.

The use of amphetamines (or "speed," in the jargon of the drug scene) has been called "the major drug-abuse problem in the U.S. outside the large cities where heroin addiction is so prevalent" in testimony before the House Select Committee on Crime. Testifying before the committee in November, 1969, Dr. George Edison, of the University of Utah, said that the amphetamines cause "dependence, physical toxicity, and behavioral toxicity." The FDA has since banned them for practically all medical uses—except the treatment of hyperkinetic children.

When the scandal exploded, there was, of course, a storm of protest from all those who, like me, consider the drugging of children shocking. Speaking on the floor of the House of Representatives the day the Washington *Post* broke the story, former Congressman Cornelius Gallagher (Democrat from New Jersey) expressed his horror and anger on learning of Omaha's drugged children. "When I read this shocking story," he told his fellow Representatives, "it seemed to me that the bright American promise of 1789 is fast turning into Huxley's brave new world in 1970."

The Congressman then went on to say: "There are many terrible and terrifying aspects to the Omaha test, but let me mention only a few at this point.

"First, the drugs employed in the Omaha test are admittedly listed by the Federal Government as dangerous substances; the FDA advises physicians to use extreme caution in prescribing one of the drugs, Ritalin, because it might lead to addiction as well as other serious side effects. Nevertheless, the drug is given in Omaha to small school-children.

"In Heaven's name, what have we come to when we use our own youngsters as guinea pigs in a grotesque game of psychological chance? Where are we heading when we administer drugs to children of six which would not be safe if given to people 10 times that age? The awful thing speaks for itself."

As a magazine editor I pitched into the battle with my own series of denunciations and accusations. There is a group of psychiatrists, I pointed out, practicing "orthomolecular psychiatry," a school that assumes many mental illnesses stem from metabolic abnormalities that prevent the patient from properly using essential nutrients like vitamins and minerals, as a result of which brain function becomes abnormal. Using very large doses of certain vitamins, notably B_3 and C, they have achieved good results even with schizophrenia. Before drugging the hyperkinetic children to modify their behavior, had the school authorities thought of investigating the children's nutritional status, I demanded, to make sure their brains had all the food they needed?

I wasn't the only questioner, of course. There was, and still is, a substantial and highly influential group insisting that hyperkinetic children really need orthomolecular treatment, while, of course, orthodox believers in psychoanalysis think it's all a question of the home environment. For all I know there may even be a transactional-analysis side in the still-raging battle. And every single viewpoint turned out to be wrong, including, I admit, the one I so ardently espoused.

What at least a good majority of hyperkinetic children—perhaps all—need is treatment for lead poisoning and a little sodium alginate in their daily diets.

As far as I can find out, the first to suspect this was Dr. Alan Cott, a New York psychiatrist. A proponent of orthomolecular therapy, he began treating hyperkinetic children with megavitamins and had some success. But he was also interested in mineral metabolism, and he decided to try a new technique, analyzing the mineral content of the hair, to make a fairly precise determination of the mineral status of the body. Dr. Cott had the hair of some of his hyperkinetic children analyzed—and found a high lead content.

He gave them the standard treatment to remove lead from the system—penicillamine, a drug closely related to penicillin. The children improved fantastically. And it began to seem as though much of the success of the megavitamin therapy was a result of the fact that the vitamins, to a limited extent, also remove a little lead from the system. Normal doses of vitamins could not remove enough to have any noticeable effect. But megavitamin doses—perhaps a hundred times larger than normal—could.

Word got around, in spite of difficulties. Most American medical journals won't publish anything unless it is already well accepted by the medical profession, so nobody ever learns anything new by reading them. When a doctor has something new and important to report, he usually does it in England.

It was in *Lancet* for October 28, 1972, that doctors Oliver David, Julian Clark and Kytja Voeller of the Departments of Psychiatry and Pediatrics of the State University of New York and Downstate Medical Center reported a careful laboratory study finding that at least 60 percent of hyperactive children examined showed excessive levels of lead in their blood. "It is concluded," they say, "that there is an association between hyperactivity and raised lead levels; that a large body-lead burden may exert consequences that have been hitherto unrealized; that the definition of what is a toxic level for blood-lead needs re-evaluation; and that physicians should look for raised levels in children with hyperactivity."

So now we begin to see why it is that the number of hyperactive and uncontrollable children in the schools is increasing year by year and why neither mood-altering drugs nor better nutrition will help most of them. What the children need is protection against lead, perhaps the most omnipresent and inescapable of all pollutants.

A danger to all of us, lead is a particular hazard to small children because they like to nibble on bits of peeled paint and plaster, both of which are likely to contain lead. This tendency for many years was known as "pica," defined as a perverted desire to eat nonfood substances. It was thought to be caused by anemia and malnutrition. Then one unorthodox and adventurous doctor actually tasted a paint flake and found it was good. Children like to eat the stuff because of its sweet flavor. (In ancient Rome lead was added to wine by storing it in lead jars, in the firm belief that it improved the flavor. Wine thus improved was very expensive and could be afforded only by the wealthiest, which may be why Caligula, Nero and many of their successors were mad, while the poor kept their balance.) In any case, at the levels of blood-lead now accepted as toxic, about 225,000 children a year are found to have excessive amounts. And David, Clark and Voeller firmly believe that the accepted level is much too high and that many more people than are known to are suffering from lead toxicity.

In November, 1972, a study was reported to the American Public Health Association meeting in Atlantic City asserting that almost one out of ten rural children examined in two neighboring New York and Connecticut counties—Dutchess and Litchfield—had unsafe amounts of lead in their blood. The study, under the direction of Professor Martha L. Lepow of the University of Connecticut Pediatrics Department, involved 230 preschool children. The findings were presented in a report, written by Dr. Lepow and Carol Cohen. It is believed to be the first time the possible dimensions of the lead-poisoning problem among rural children has been assessed.

In her sample of one-, two- and five-year-old children, Miss Cohen found that 20 (9 percent) had unsafe amounts of lead in their blood. This contrasted with a 1971 sample of urban youngsters in Hartford which showed 22 percent had lead traces above the safe limits. The rural children had more than 40 micrograms of lead per 100 milliliters of blood, or 0.4 parts per million, the maximum "safe" level set by the U.S. Surgeon General, which is very likely far too high.

Other facts of the study: The average amount of blood-lead for each of the 230 rural children stood at 22.8 micrograms of lead per 100 milliliters of blood, or 0.228 parts per million, a quantity defined as "safe" today but quite possibly on the borderline of danger.

Only 2 percent of the 230 children came from "welfare" families.

More than nine in ten were white—91 percent.

The father was head of the household for 89 percent of the families.

About 70 percent of the children were from families in the two lowest socioeconomic classes, as ranked by education and occupation.

As is common with urban studies of lead poisoning, most of the rural children with elevated blood-lead levels lived in housing more than twenty-five years old, where flaking lead-based paint or plaster was common.

However, lead poisoning is far from being something that happens only to children in the slums who eat sweet-tasting paint chips from the walls of their tenement apartments. The parents of three-year-old Joshua Guenter and two-year-old Natasha Babayan, among many others, know better. They are middle-class people, living in comfortable Manhattan brownstone homes which they carefully cleared of all lead-based paint. To their horror, however, a New York Health Department survey found in 1972 that without eating a single paint chip their children had levels of lead in their blood dangerously close to the amount shown to cause damage. They were lucky—their children's problem was detected in time to save them from dangerous lead poisoning.

We're all victims—or potential victims—of lead poisoning. Most of us don't show obvious signs, yet we're each exposed to terrifying quantities of lead every day, in the air we breathe, in the food we eat and the water we drink, and in other, less conspicuous sources such as improperly glazed pottery. The biggest enemy is that automobile sitting in your driveway. In fact, the National Air Pollution Control Administration estimates that 200,000 tons of lead are added to the atmosphere each year and that 95 percent of that massive dose of poison comes from automobile exhaust. And, despite television commercials you see hailing "no-lead" and "low-lead" gasolines, a test reported in the Washington *Post* (June 12, 1971) shows that even the lowest of the "no-lead" gasolines averages .046 grams of lead per gallon.

Lead is a nonessential, poisonous element. We don't need—and shouldn't have—*any* of it in our systems. But it's practically inescapable. So inescapable, in fact, that "normal" levels have been established. Supposedly, if your blood lead remains below a certain point (some authorities suggest 0.2 parts per million, half the official safe level), you won't show any signs of lead poisoning.

However, when your blood lead rises above the "acceptable" level, your system can be seriously upset. In adults, sufficient quantities can cause fatigue, sleep disturbances, lack of appetite and constipation, in the early stages. Doctors, unfortunately, often attribute these symptoms to that catch-all, "the virus." And, says Dr. J. Julian Chisolm, one of the country's foremost experts on lead poisoning, once your blood-lead level rises above "normal," your system slows down its excretion of the poison, letting it accumulate in even greater concentrations. As the concentration of lead builds, anemia, "lead-lines" in your bones (lead accumulates there), irritability and confusion evidence themselves, and kidney damage, convulsions, paralysis, blindness, sterility and even death may occur. In addition, lead in the air is beginning to cause abnormalities in our body chemistry, according to Dr. Henry A. Schroeder of Dartmouth Medical School's Trace Elements Laboratory.

For expectant mothers, lead is even more dangerous. Children born to lead-poisoned women, a report from the Environmental Health Service states, suffer growth retardation, survival problems after birth and nervous-system spasms. The report adds that lead poisoning "frequently causes sterility or early spontaneous abortion."

Between the air, the food, the water and the numerous other exposures to lead we suffer each day, the metal appears to be inescapable. And forcing your child to live in a lead-polluted world is cruel and unusual punishment. Children are far more susceptible to the poison than adults. Besides hyperactivity and the early, so-called minor, symptoms which adults suffer, children can undergo permanent brain damage, mental retardation, blindness and abnormal behavior development. A recent report by Professor

Derek Bryce-Smith of the University of Reading in England suggests that the increasing rates of admission to mental hospitals in Britain can be credited to the increasing amounts of lead in our environment (*New Scientist and Science Journal,* June 27, 1971). The effects of lead poisoning on children are so depressing, in fact, that Roger Caras, in an article entered in the *Congressional Record* (June 14, 1971), writes: "Lead eaten by a child can result in death. Perhaps those that die are among the lucky ones, for many of those that survive are afflicted with everything from loss of sight to severe mental retardation."

Unlike mercury and DDT, lead as a poison generally has not been brought to the public attention, and has not excited the protests of the public, except in the case of lead paint on the walls of slum apartments. This is a step in the right direction, for, according to a story in the *New York Times* (October 10, 1970), "a piece of paint the size of a thumb nail—eaten 3 times a week over a period of several months—can make a child sick." But this still is not enough. Joshua Guenter and Natasha Babayan did not eat paint from the wall—they merely breathed the air.

The simple fact is that every revolution of every auto engine burning leaded gasoline sprays the atmosphere with tiny particles of lead oxide. In city streets where there is a heavy concentration of traffic, children like Joshua and Natasha are actually accumulating toxic concentrations of lead simply from the air they breathe. And even in the country, where traffic is not so heavy, there are periodic alarms over lead residues on food crops, also stemming from the exhaust pipes of automobiles.

Of course our cars have emission controls, and are supposed to emit no lead at all by 1976. But nobody believes the requirement will be met. And to date all tests have shown that, even if an emission-control system works fine when a car is new, it is practically ineffective after the car has been driven a few thousand miles. And the lead from the cars settles everywhere—in our water, on the food in markets, on the dishes we eat from. Vegetables from gardens in a town of nine thousand population in New York State showed over one hundred parts per million of lead.

One would guess that even the Environmental Protection Agency does not expect emission-control regulations to alleviate the lead problem from the fact that the agency has quietly gone to McGill University with funding for a study to find a way to remove lead from the body. You will recall it was the Gastrointestinal Research Laboratory of McGill that was successful in finding a nontoxic readily available material—sodium alginate—that is so effective in removing radioactive strontium from the body it will actually be of use in a fallout emergency.

Again under the direction of Dr. Stanley Skoryna, the lab went into the new problem as exhaustively as it had tackled its predecessor. And, miracle of miracles, they emerged from their study with exactly the same answer.

Sodium alginate, they found, will do a better job of removing lead from the body than any other known material. In the case of lead, it will even be removed slowly from the blood, while everything accumulated in the digestive system will of course be carried away. That added effect comes about because lead tends to circulate in the blood for a long while before it is finally deposited in the bones. While the blood is circulating, it passes through the intestines over and over again; and each time, if there is any of the chelating material in the gut, it will leach some of the lead out of the blood.

When you think of 225,000 children a year, or more, accumulating excessive lead in their systems, threatened with brain damage, unable to learn properly, feeling fatigue, nausea, possibly having all their potential destroyed, then I think you will agree that learning how to incorporate this nonnutritive but useful ingredient into recipes is as important a task as any mother can face.

One easy way to do it is suggested in the journal *Environmental Research* for October, 1971, in a paper by K. Kostial and associates of the Institute for Medical Research of the Yugoslav Academy of Arts and Sciences. The Yugoslav scientists found that adding alginates to milk will actually induce a substantial increase in the amount of lead removed from the system, as compared with alginates alone. Adding a little alginate powder to milk simply thickens it a little, without changing the flavor in any way. The milk itself, as you may have guessed, also plays a role in getting rid of lead, because of its high calcium content.

One of the most important of recent studies, carried out by Dr. Kathryn M. Six and Dr. Robert A. Goyer of the University of North Carolina, and reported to the 1971 meeting of the Federation of American Societies for Experimental Biology, demonstrated that large quantities of calcium in the diet exert a strong preventive effect on the damage lead can do while, conversely, a low-calcium diet permits the full toxic effects of lead to occur.

What Dr. Six and Dr. Goyer did was to experiment with a group of albino rats, an animal whose reactions to lead are very close to those of human beings. The rats were fed on varying diets containing calcium to a level of .9 percent. At the level of slightly less than 1 percent calcium, it was shown that a given level of two hundred parts per million of lead acetate in the drinking water will not produce any significant changes in the size or function of the kidneys or in the ability of the animals under study to generate new blood as needed. That in itself is a highly significant discovery. To achieve a calcium level of nearly 1 percent of the total diet would be difficult for anybody, but by no means impossible to those determined to do it. It would take a strong concentration of green, leafy vegetables in the diet and then, of course, plenty of milk and perhaps further supplementation with calcium.

Having established the level of calcium intake that would neutralize the effects of two hundred parts per million of lead in drinking water, Dr. Six and Dr. Goyer then proceeded to find out what would happen to the experimental animals at lower levels of calcium intake. Using as controls a group of animals that drank lead-free distilled water, they fed both groups diets containing less than .9 percent of calcium, in varying percentages, dropping as low as .1 percent. After ten weeks of this feeding the animals were sacrificed and intensively examined. As described in *Nutrition Reviews* (June, 1971): "The animals receiving lead in their drinking water showed a greater absorption of lead when the dietary calcium was low. At the upper level of calcium intake there were greater amounts of lead recovered in the feces."

The blood level of lead was found to be four times as high in the animals receiving the low-calcium diet. The animals on the low-calcium diet had also suffered a marked increase in kidney size compared to those given larger amounts of calcium; all showed symptoms of lead poisoning, compared to only two out of seven of the group with the .9 percent calcium intake. The authors concluded that the less calcium there is in the diet, the more lead will be absorbed into the system.

Another significant piece of research was performed by Dr. E. D. Hobart and associates at Rush Medical College in Chicago. It was reported to the 1971 Chicago meeting of the Federation of American Societies for Experimental Biology. Dr. Hobart showed that vitamin C can have an important role in protecting muscle tissue from lead damage. Working with guinea pigs, Dr. Hobart and his fellow scientists fed a diet containing .25 percent lead to animals deficient in vitamin C. The result: widespread damage of muscle fiber and calcium deposits around the damaged cells. Vitamin C, they point out, is essential in producing the tissue which connects the muscle fibers (connective tissue). Too much lead and too little vitamin C can produce disastrous results.

We don't synthesize vitamin C in our bodies, and therefore must take a sufficient amount each day to replenish our capacity to resist the effects of lead. And our systems can't store vitamin C for long periods of time, so it's best to replenish the stores of it several times each day. We get it by eating plenty of cabbage, tomatoes, fresh fruits (especially cantaloupe, apples and strawberries), broccoli, green peppers and citrus fruits and then by taking supplements of the vitamin. It is worthwhile. It will not remove any lead from your body, but it *will* reduce the damage.

Finally, even though we know a good way to protect ourselves against environmental lead, it still does no harm to exercise some care and avoid lead whenever we can. Washing all vegetables carefully before using them can remove a good bit of the auto-exhaust lead that settles on their surfaces. It will help to keep your car windows closed when driving in very heavy traffic—particularly in tunnels. If you live on a heavy-traffic street, you should also keep your windows closed at home. Most importantly, be careful about the dishes you eat from. One of the commonest causes of acute lead poisoning is lead-containing glazes on earthenware.

One case reported in the AMA *Journal* concerned a fifty-five-year-old doctor who didn't understand this danger well enough to avoid it. He suffered from generalized fatigue, a feeling of heaviness in his arms, insomnia, headaches, lack of appetite, nausea and occasional loose stools. He lost ten pounds in a single month. Crampy abdominal pains had lasted several weeks before he entered the hospital. A week of testing disclosed that the patient was suffering from lead poisoning so severe that even after two weeks of hospitalization, with presumed total absence from exposure to source, the level of lead in the blood remained dangerously high. It took three months of therapy with a calcium compound to get the concentration of lead out of the urine and blood.

That out of the way, the hunt was on for the cause. The *Journal of the American Medical Association* (November 6, 1967) reports that questioning at first seemed futile, "but the patient's wife soon offered a key clue to the mystery. It seems that the patient had the unique habit of filling a ceramic mug, made by his son, with ice and a soft drink. He sipped the chilled soda during a period of several hours in the evening, usually refilling the mug with a second bottle of cola. This had been an almost nightly ritual for the two years preceding his admission to the hospital."

The mug was examined at a laboratory, and tests showed that over 5 milligrams of lead were leached from the mug for every 450 cubic centimeters of cola within half an hour.

Dr. Robert W. Harris and Dr. William R. Elsea described the mug as a yellow ceramic, with smooth glazed outer finish, and the inside quite faded and chalky. When Harris and Elsea filled the cup with cola, there was a rapid appearance of lead in the soft drink. This did not happen when the cup was filled with water. The acidity of the soft drink reacted with the lining of the cup and released the lead. The doctor's son had enrolled in a ceramics class at college and molded several mugs identical to the one he gave his father. His was one of the few classes to use lead oxide as a glazing agent. The students were told about the dangers of handling lead glazes, but nobody was concerned about the use of the articles.

When the authors reviewed the literature on lead poisoning, it became evident that this situation was not unusual. Numerous experiences with acidic food and drink and lead-glazed utensils were noted in the past, at least as far back as the Roman Empire. And as recently as 1967 a gastrointestinal epidemic in Mexico was blamed on poorly fired lead-glazed earthenware. The AMA *Journal* story warns that "the popularity of ceramics as an art and hobby, and paucity of government regulations would seem certainly to offer a potentially dangerous situation, considering that the ceramics industry uses 25,000 to 30,000 tons of lead a year." In California recently an entire family suffered lead poisoning because they drank fruit juice from a highly artistic pottery pitcher.

It could happen to anyone who isn't aware. And while sodium alginate and calcium can give you very good protection, you're still better off to avoid taking lead into your body. It's the only protection that is 100 percent effective.

13 There's Death in Your Garage

Nearly fifty years ago, when I was a boy, I had my first experience with death. In a typical gasoline alley—an alley lined on both sides with one-car garages—I saw a group of neighbors drag a man out of his garage. His face was bright red and there was a froth of bloody bubbles around his mouth. Attempts to revive him by artificial respiration failed.

He was killed by carbon monoxide, an invisible, odorless gas that is constantly pouring out of the exhaust pipe of every car in the world whenever its engine runs. Unlike lead and polycyclic hydrocarbons, whose poisonous nature when emitted from tailpipes has been learned relatively recently, the fact that the carbon-monoxide emission can kill people has been known almost as long as there have been cars. Yet nothing has ever been done about it, except for warnings from various sages that it is unwise to run your engine in a closed garage. Emission controls do not yet reduce the amount of carbon monoxide being poured into the air. Factories, incinerators and power plants get their chimneys equipped with elaborate filters to trap solid particles from their smoke emissions, but they make no effort to reduce the carbon monoxide. We are pouring this poison gas into the air in really incredible quantities. At a Conference on Biological Effects of

Carbon Monoxide in New York in January, 1970, it was stated that ninety-four million tons of this poison gas were emitted in the United States in the year 1966. It is worse today, of course. Today there are more cars—almost one hundred million in operation in the United States—and cars are responsible for some 75 percent of the carbon monoxide in the air.

For a long time carbon monoxide was considered harmless once it was dispersed into the outside air but now it has accumulated to such levels that it is coming to be recognized as an important cause of ill health and even death. Careful charts of the relationship have been kept by the California Department of Public Health, and it was well explored in an article by Alfred C. Hexster and John R. Goldsmith of that department published in *Science* for April 16, 1971. Comparing carbon-monoxide concentrations with the number of deaths in Los Angeles for every day of the four-year period 1962–1965, these Public Health statisticians found that on any day when the carbon-monoxide concentration in the air reaches as much as twenty parts per million, there are eleven more deaths than would otherwise occur. They believe, on the basis of evidence published in the *Archives of Environmental Health* (19, 510; 1969) by S. I. Cohen and co-workers, that these extra deaths are due to heart attack and are so classified in the mortality statistics.

It is really not hard to see why.

Carbon monoxide is about 56 percent oxygen, which is enough to permit it to act like oxygen in some respects. When it is inhaled, it passes through the lungs into the bloodstream just as oxygen does. Normally a red cell of the blood passing through the lungs will pick up a molecule of oxygen, which it will carry to the heart and then to the other tissues of the body, the oxygen being drawn away by any tissue cell that comes in contact with it and happens to need it. But if, in the lungs, the red cell contacts a molecule of carbon monoxide rather than pure oxygen, it is the carbon monoxide that is picked up. The tissues cannot use carbon monoxide so they don't remove it from the red cells. The blood keeps circulating with its red cells unable to get rid of the carbon-monoxide molecules and therefore unable to pick up oxygen molecules.

If one breathes enough carbon monoxide to inactivate a critical number of red blood cells, the result is anoxia—lack of oxygen—and possibly death. More than a thousand people a year die of this acute carbon-monoxide poisoning.

An unknown number of people die because a carbon-monoxide-induced reduction in the supply of oxygen to the heart causes myocardial infarction, the death of heart tissue through oxygen starvation.

In a study of 3,080 case histories from 36 Los Angeles County hospitals, there was a 27.3 death rate for patients who lived in high-carbon-monoxide zones. But in "low pollution areas, deaths averaged 19.1 in 100."

In a small farming community north of Tokyo Dr. Tomio Komatu reports seasonal results of carbon-monoxide poisoning. A local health officer, Dr. Komatu observed that each spring 33 percent of the 2,000 inhabitants of the small community exhibited swollen faces and hands; chronic heart disease and rheumatism were also prevalent, with about 40 percent of the deaths from cardiac causes, he told the *Mainichi Daily News* (April 5, 1972) in an interview. Dr. Komatu's investigation revealed that these people spent the winter months "processing hemp fibers in poorly ventilated rooms, heated with open charcoal fireboxes. The carbon monoxide concentration in the air under these conditions averaged 70 parts per million and in some rooms reached 200 parts per million. A concentration of 100 parts per million is sufficient to provoke symptoms of acute carbon monoxide poisoning."

There are also other results for those who do not breathe enough carbon monoxide to be killed. For the past few years studies have been conducted on the influence of low levels of carboxyhemoglobin, with particular interest directed at cigarette smokers.

Dr. John Goldsmith and Dr. Seymour Landau told the 1970 Conference on Biological Effects of Carbon Monoxide that CO is a major contributor to motor-vehicle accidents. They said studies suggest "that drivers with high levels of carbon monoxide in their blood may be more prone to accidents" (*Health News,* March, 1969). This was borne out in two recent studies at Ohio State University. Drivers, accompanied by a physician and a research engineer, were given CO until their blood levels reached 10 to 20 percent. The subjects were put through a number of tests before and after the gas was administered. They did not know they were being given carbon monoxide. The tests included estimating time and distance, discriminating tail-light brightness on the car they were following, and estimating the speed of their own car as well as the vehicle being followed.

The effect of increased carbon monoxide was apparent on all the performance tests. Researchers found the greatest effect was in response time and the driver's judgment. Of note, too, was the increased fatigue felt by the subjects after trying to stay in the middle of their lane for ten minutes at a speed of sixty-five miles per hour. These and other studies suggest that many highway accidents—particularly one-car accidents—are caused by fatigue and drowsiness aggravated by carbon monoxide, which can easily enter the passenger compartment from a defective muffler. Deprived of oxygen, the body is actually in a state of deterioration—in effect, the body is a little bit dead.

Another highly significant way that carbon monoxide can and does contribute to automobile accidents was revealed in Denver in January, 1973, at a Conference of the American College of Chest Physicians. Dr. Wilbert S. Aronow of the University of California at Irvine told the Conference that exposure to highway traffic on heavily traveled expressways for ninety minutes had been found to bring on symptoms of angina pectoris in some drivers and passengers.

Two sets of freeway studies were performed. In the first, the subjects were driven in station wagons with windows open during heavy early-morning freeway traffic for ninety minutes. Each subject had been fitted with a miniaturized, continuously recording electrocardiograph. In the second study, three weeks later, the same procedure was repeated except that the car windows were closed and the patients breathed purified compressed air through masks. Blood tests showed that driving in heavy traffic with open windows raised the level of carbon monoxide in the blood from 5.4 parts per million to 21.5 parts per million. Two hours after the test had concluded, the blood level was still 13.6 parts per million.

Such an accumulation, we have already seen, could be expected to lead to drowsiness, loss of coordination, dulled responses and impaired judgment of time and distance. And those effects will obviously greatly reduce a driver's chances of being able to stay out of a crash. But the induction of symptoms of angina pectoris makes the situation far worse.

Angina, which is brought on by an insufficient oxygen supply to the heart, is both painful and frightening. It is a crushing pain that occurs suddenly in the chest. Although it is not a heart attack, it feels as though it could be. The person who suffers an attack has a tendency to double over and press his hands and arms to his chest. You can imagine the effect of that when you're driving a car at sixty-five miles an hour on a freeway.

So it may readily be seen that, even though there are not many numbers to go by, carbon monoxide is and must be an important cause of automobile accidents. In most cases it is surely overlooked as the cause. The gas has no odor, no taste and no color. Detection without instruments is impossible. The effect is slow and subtle and you are not warned by tearing eyes or spasms of coughing. Vision dims gradually and perhaps imperceptibly. A throbbing headache may never be blamed on carbon monoxide. You feel drowsy but don't doubt that you can manage to stay awake. Crash. Do you end up dead or merely maimed?

In 1973 the number of deaths in the United States caused by

automobile accidents since such statistics have been recorded reached two million. How many were the effect of carbon-monoxide pollution?

I think I must have made my point that it's desirable to protect yourself against carbon monoxide in all circumstances, but particularly when driving your car. The question is, what can you do about it?

First, let's understand clearly that if you're going to close your garage door on a cold or rainy day while you tinker with your carburetor, or if you're going to heat a closed vacation cabin with an unvented stove, there's nothing you can do. You're going to be asphyxiated and there is no measure known that is going to protect you against that kind of folly.

On the other hand, however, your normal problem as a driver is to counteract the effect of relatively low though toxic concentrations of carbon monoxide in the atmosphere. Of course you're going to have your muffler checked frequently and make sure it isn't leaking into the passenger compartment. So we don't have to worry about that.

The most important internal protection you can give yourself is to make sure that you never allow yourself to become anemic, and in fact have blood of better than average rich redness. The redder your blood, the more red cells it contains and the greater the content of hemoglobin, the special material that enables red cells to transport oxygen, in each cell. Remember that carbon monoxide does its damage by putting out of commission enough red blood cells to reduce the supply of oxygen to the tissues. The more such cells you have in your blood, the more carbon monoxide it will take to affect you, and the longer it will take for any traffic concentration of the gas to do you damage. So if you are one of the many millions who are compelled to drive daily for long periods of time in heavy traffic, perhaps through tunnels which are far worse than the Los Angeles freeways, it might be very well to have your doctor check the condition of your blood.

A surprising number of readers are going to find that they are anemic, particularly those who are female. If your doctor does find a frank anemia, he will of course treat it. There is a very good chance, however, that he will tell you something like: "It's a little low but nothing to worry about," or "Perfectly normal for a woman," or the equivalent verdict indicating that your blood hemoglobin content is within the range recognized as normal, but that there is definite room for improvement. In such a case your doctor doesn't want to bother with iron injections because they are rather painful and can have some unpleasant side effects.

It would not be very difficult under optimal circumstances for people to get the needed 0.5 to 1 milligram of iron daily straight from their diets, and, in fact, the average man can do so with no problems. According to the AMA Council on Foods and Nutrition, the person least likely to be affected by iron deficiency is the adult male, who requires 3.5 grams if he weighs 154 pounds. About 70 percent of that iron is actually being used; the other 30 percent is stored for emergencies. If the man takes 0.5 to 1 milligram of iron in his diet daily, he ought to be able to maintain his iron balance, with a constant store of 3.5 grams or more.

The average woman, however, has less iron in her body than the average man, 2.3 grams, while ideally she ought to have as much as a man. But there is a whole host of factors which can interfere with a woman's ability to meet all of her iron needs through the ordinary diet. Once a girl reaches adolescence and begins menstruating, for example, she loses significantly higher levels of blood than a man ordinarily does. Since over 80 percent of the iron in her body is found in the red cells of the blood, loss of the blood through menstruation also means a significant loss of iron. Dr. L. Hallberg reported in *Acta Obstetrica Gynecologica Scandinavica* (45: 1966), that iron loss in menstruating women is about 0.5 milligrams per day. Other researchers have estimated that the loss could be from 0.7 to 2 milligrams per day. That loss in itself is between two and four times the needed daily intake for the average man.

Pregnant women need even more iron. Especially during the last four months of pregnancy, iron is transferred to the fetus and the placenta in large amounts. When the baby is born, the mother loses significant amounts of iron through blood loss. In addition, a pregnant woman's body produces about 30 percent more red blood cells than it normally would—and such production requires a great deal of iron. All this boils down to an iron requirement of up to 7.5 milligrams daily during the last six months of pregnancy. According to the AMA position paper on iron deficiency, "The required amounts are beyond the amount available from diet. Iron stores are frequently absent in pregnancy. In women with depleted stores, supplemental iron therapy during the last half of pregnancy is essential if iron deficiency is to be prevented." Lactation also uses iron, and the loss to a woman who is nursing her baby is approximately 0.5 to 1 milligram daily.

Certain disease conditions can also use up iron. An apparently mild bleeding ulcer can cause significant blood losses over a period of years—and iron losses as a consequence.

The average American diet provides 6 milligrams of iron per 1,000 calories. And the average caloric intake for a woman somewhat interested in weight control is 1,500 to 2,000. The normal man may eat as many as 3,000 calories a day. Thus, for most people, iron intake ranges from 12 to 18 milligrams daily.

That seems like more than enough to meet the average person's daily needs. It isn't, however, because only a small percentage of the iron we eat is absorbed into the body. Less than 10 percent of the iron stored in vegetables is ever used by the body, and about 20 percent of animal-protein iron is useful. Thus, your body probably absorbs a good deal less than 2 milligrams of iron per day from the food you eat.

The average man, if he is not a frequent blood donor, will probably get by on that. The average woman will not. According to the AMA, "Present limitations in iron intake also justify further fortification of the diet for menstruating women. While there is inadequate information concerning iron deficiency and iron deficiency anemia in this segment of the population, frequent iron depletion is found when marrow iron stores are examined. Thus Scott and Pritchard (*Journal of the American Medical Association,* March 20, 1967) found scant to absent iron stores in 66 of 114 menstruating women, and Monsen (*American Journal of Clinical Nutrition,* August, 1967) found absent stores in 9 of 13 women studied. Furthermore, absence of iron stores in the majority of pregnant women in their third trimester, necessitating the medicinal therapy, is a clear indication of the inadequate stores with which most women enter pregnancy."

If inadequate for the normal demands of pregnancy, or simply of being a woman, how much more so for the problem of keeping the blood at peak condition to maximize the oxygen supply, even when in an atmosphere heavily laden with carbon monoxide. You will obviously want to do what you can to enrich your blood in the course of day-to-day living. The way to do it is to eat better.

The first common-sense step is to increase your intake of foods rich in iron. These include liver and other meats, parsley, lettuce and other greens and wheat germ.

The well-known Harvard nutritionist Jean Mayer, stressing the importance of diet in combating iron deficiency, wrote in the November, 1968, issue of *Postgraduate Medicine,* "This [a good diet] is all the more important at a time when iron cooking utensils have been eliminated, thus eliminating an appreciable source of iron in the diet, when fat represents over 40 per cent of the American diet, and when dietary products (extremely low in iron) are consumed in large amounts. The U.S. diet is often much lower in iron than are the diets of poorer populations, which are high in partially milled cereals prepared in primitive pots and pans."

Dr. Mayer has no faith in modern-day foods to meet the great need for iron, especially in women. He says, "While we can hope that women will eat some meat, fish, eggs and green vegetables, it is unrealistic to hope that they will eat the frequent portions of liver which women with copious menstrual losses require. Once anemia has set in, it is unrealistic to think it can be cured by diet alone."

There is, however, one easy and painless way to get more liver into your diet, and that is to use supplements of what is known as desiccated liver. The rather unattractive name designates a powder that is pure beef liver, reduced by drying to about one-fourth the bulk. It contains the iron content of four times the weight of cooked liver. You can get it in tablets so that you can swallow your liver without even tasting it, if you happen to hate liver. But perhaps the best way to take it is by adding a tablespoon of the powder to a soup, a gravy or a glass of tomato juice.

Taking your desiccated liver with tomato juice might be especially helpful, since it has been pointed out by the English nutritionist Dr. John Marks that "there is experimental evidence that ascorbic acid (vitamin C) is a factor in the formation of hemoglobin." There is also a recent clinical study described in *Nutrition Reports International* for December, 1971, showing that adequate vitamin C, on the order of two to three hundred milligrams a day, is necessary for optimal hemoglobin formation. And still other studies have shown that the amount of iron absorbed from food is increased by 30 percent if it is accompanied by vitamin C in the same meal.

So the combination of desiccated liver and tomato juice has a lot going for it and should serve, if taken daily, to provide your body with a good reserve of iron and your blood with a high level of red cells to transport oxygen—enough to keep you normal even if carbon monoxide puts 5 percent of them temporarily out of commission.

There are also a couple of other measures you can take to try to reduce the amount of CO you are compelled to breathe.

One is simply to close your car windows.

Now we are customarily warned never to ride with our windows closed completely, because the muffler may have a hole in it, and if it does, it could leak CO into the passenger compartment. That's perfectly correct. It's the advice to follow if you're not sure about the condition of your muffler—if you don't *know* beyond a doubt that your muffler is good.

But, now that you know as much as you do about the dangers of CO, I must presume that the very least you are going to do about it is have your muffler checked frequently. If you know it's in good condition, before you drive into that daily traffic jam on the Schuylkill Expressway or the West Side Highway or the San Diego Freeway, shut your windows and keep out that traffic-jam air that is just loaded with CO, lead and other poisonous emissions. Driving through the Holland Tunnel with your windows open is foolhardy courage, like volunteering for the paratroops.

Another good rule is not to smoke while driving, especially in heavy traffic.

If you're a cigarette smoker, you may be familiar with those times when your face gets red, your vision becomes a little blurry, and you become aware that your mind just isn't working right. That's all a result of the carbon monoxide that is in cigarette smoke, and indeed in all products of all combustion. Two cigarettes will put as much carbon monoxide into your blood as an hour in fairly heavy traffic.

Both smoking and carbon monoxide are undesirable, but together they are twice as undesirable. If you smoke in heavy traffic you are really courting an oxygen shortage that can lead to an accident or a heart attack.

And lastly, as an emergency measure, there is oxygen. Oxygen is the standard medical therapy for CO poisoning, according to the *Merck Manual,* that little handbook your doctor keeps out of sight in the room behind his office and is consulting when he excuses himself for a minute.

If you want to prepare for a possible situation in which CO pollution will be both unavoidable and severe, like a bus breakdown in the Lincoln Tunnel in rush hour, you can buy a small cylinder of 70 percent oxygen in many drugstores. If you start to feel flushed and drowsy, sitting in a sea of idling and overheating cars, you can take a couple of whiffs of oxygen and improve the situation.

It is a dangerous remedy. Too much oxygen can do almost as much harm as too little. It might put you in a kind of drunken state in which you will laugh or giggle and lose all your judgment. It is also a highly flammable gas that can be ignited by any strong spark. In fact, there is enough danger in self-administration of oxygen to have made me hesitate even to mention it. There are, however, those occasional situations where the CO levels are mounting and inescapable and, particularly if you have a bad heart, you can feel the bad air doing you in. Oxygen, in such a situation, can be a lifesaver. But don't abuse it. That's risky.

14 Stay Alert to Stay Alive

What is a pollutant? It is something inimical to health and life that has been added to the environment by man. Can you think of a better description of the automobile?

To my mind the automobile is the greatest hazard in our environment. It kills fifty to sixty thousand people a year, injures and maims two million more. And these figures do not take into account the lead, cadmium, carbon monoxide and polycyclic hydrocarbons that motor vehicles pour into the air.

Perhaps because it is gross rather than microscopic, perhaps because we feel we are in control of whether our cars are destroyers or merely transportation, you may not agree that the car is actually a pollutant. That is your privilege. Indisputably, however, it is the greatest single hazard in our environment. On the assumption that you wouldn't be reading this book if you didn't want to stay alive with a sound body, I'd like to pass along some information you probably don't have to improve your chances. There's really a lot more to safe driving than just buckling your seat belt. The real trick is to stay out of accidents completely. And a great deal of your success in doing so will depend on your own muscle tone.

During the past twelve months, chances are someone you know

was involved in an auto accident. Whoever he was, he blamed the other guy, or a bad curve in the road, or a blind intersection, or an unsafe automobile. If he is like most of us, it was absolutely "not his fault."

The uncomfortable truth, charges British industrialist T. S. Skillman, in his book *How To Reduce Road Accidents* (The Re-Appraisal Society, London, 1965) is that "It is the ordinary driver who is the chief cause of accidents—there are no safe drivers."

More than seven hundred physicians, nurses and medical students reached substantially that same conclusion in 1972 when they voted on what they considered to be the chief cause of driving accidents. According to 79 percent of the voting delegates at the Texas Medical Convention, poor driver reflexes are the single most important factor in causing crashes.

Say you're driving down Main Street at thirty miles an hour. Forty feet in front of you, without warning, a parked car pulls into your lane. Naturally, you slam on the brake.

But, if it takes you as little as one second to get the message from your eyeballs to your brain that the car has cut you off, and another message from your brain to your foot to get off the gas and on the brake, the stop you come to will be four feet into the other guy's fender. For at thirty miles an hour you are traveling forty-four feet every second.

And that doesn't mean you will bring your car to a dead stop in a second, or forty-four feet. Even if you press the brake pedal through the floorboard, the car can skid another fifty-six feet before inertia is overcome—unless it hits another vehicle first.

Let's say you are ripping along on an expressway at sixty miles an hour. Then, it will take you 366 feet to bring your car to a stop. Eighty-eight of those feet are spent getting your foot to the brake. Last Christmas, a twenty-two-year-old college student was on his way home from a small school in Westchester, New York. Traveling along one of the winding ice-covered roads near the Palisades, he saw a car in the oncoming lane tear around a curve at breakneck speed and skid out of control. Instantly the young man drove into a snowbank, spun around, and still traveling toward the oncoming car, hit the snowbank again with the rear bumper. His car finally came to a halt four feet from the other car.

That boy's life was saved by a quarter of a second in reaction time.

Reaction time in its very technical sense is the period from a stimulus—seeing the car skid out of control into your lane, for example—to the very beginning of the physical response—lifting the foot off the gas and turning the wheel. That reaction time is basically inherited and cannot be improved upon to any great extent.

In normal people, it may range from slightly over one-tenth of a second to as much as a quarter of a second, according to Joseph B. Oxendine, professor and chairman of the Department of Health, Physical Education and Recreation at Temple University. Contrary to general opinion, pure reaction time does not vary greatly with age. Grandfather's reactions are likely to be just as fast as junior's.

Where grandfather will probably have to yield to the younger generation is in "movement" time, the period from when the foot leaves the accelerator to when it is pressed firmly down on the brake. In driving, that phase is invariably more time-consuming than the actual reaction. If it takes as little as one second, your car going at thirty miles an hour will travel forty-four feet before the brakes will begin to slow it down.

Pure reaction time you can't control—you're either fast or you're slow—and the difference between the two extremes amounts to about one-seventh of a second. But what you can control to a significant extent is your movement time. With a little effort, even grandfather could probably cut his movement time clear in half, and give junior a run for his money. According to Professor Oxendine, "The movement phase of reaction speed is based on muscular force, and is therefore modifiable through practicing and conditioning." Exercise, in other words, can significantly cut the amount of time it takes you to respond behind the wheel. If actual movement time is to be decreased, "exercise movements exactly like driving would be best," Oxendine says. The idea is to strengthen precisely those muscles which are required for specific movement in driving.

As most teenagers learned ages ago, a light, sporty car with a powerful engine will accelerate much faster than Dad's heavy family car with an average-sized engine. Power (or strength) and speed are tied together.

The stronger your arm and leg muscles are, the faster they can move ten or twenty pounds of flesh in response to your brain's commands. Want to cut your movement time by up to 50 percent? Here are some exercises to improve the condition of precisely those muscles you are going to have to use when you get into an emergency situation in your car.

Bicycling. While lying on your back, lift your feet about thirty inches off the floor. Begin a bicycle-pedaling motion, and maintain it until the fatigue is considerable. Rest for a minute and repeat.

Do not pedal rapidly. Extend the foot all the way, then pull the knee back at least as far as the waist. The goal is to establish muscle fatigue, for muscle strength does not begin to develop until fatigue is encountered.

Muscles can also be strengthened by actual bicycle riding. Make sure you use leg muscle to push the pedals down, rather than standing over them using your weight to propel them. Dr. Oxendine considers this a very good exercise for decreasing movement time.

Weight training. Two ten-pound dumbbells will go a long way toward helping you to build arm muscles for steering faster in emergencies. With one in each hand, keeping palms toward the floor, make circular motions. Again, the number of circles depends on your own endurance. Keep going for several circles past the time when it begins to hurt. Then rest for a minute.

Hold the weights in front of you, your palms facing each other and the upper arms flat against your sides. Lift the weights slowly in vertical parallels. Afterward, rotate them in half circles.

Half knee bends. Knee bends can be combined effectively with the weight training exercises. Be sure to keep your back vertical rather than inclined forward, since that position more closely approximates your posture while driving. It is not necessary to do as deep a knee bend as you did in your salad days. Go as far as you can without throwing anything out of joint.

You can invent additional exercises which will fit your daily schedule and preferences. As you build your personal program remember that the exercises must involve the precise muscles used in driving reactions—and they must be stressed the same way they would be while driving.

A final word about fast reactions. Quick responses require alertness. If your mind wanders for just a few seconds, you can travel hundreds of feet before reaction, movement and braking come into play.

Exercise is important here, too. Professor Oxendine says that keeping the body generally fit does make one more alert—and a number of studies indicate that high school and college students who are physically fit perform better academically too. Any exercises which stimulate the entire body and circulatory system help to promote alertness. Jogging is good. So are swimming, tennis and volleyball. For those badly out of condition, a brisk walk daily is perhaps all that should be attempted.

Never underestimate the importance of alertness. If, while you're driving, you notice your concentration is not up to par, pull off the road. If you are drowsy, rest. If not, then get some exercise. Walk around the car, do bending and stretching exercises. The blood will flow faster as the heart beats harder. Fresh oxygen in large quantities will be carried by the blood to the brain, and that will help make you more alert.

Alertness, of course, can involve a great deal more than just the tone of our muscles. We have all been warned so often about drinking when driving that it would be pointless to repeat the warnings here, even though they are perfectly correct. Did you know, however, that marijuana, which is regarded by many people as a stimulant, has also been found to slow a driver's response time?

There has been a great deal of discussion about this, pro and con, reflecting chiefly the prejudices of law-abiding non-users and the folklore of popular music, many of whose practitioners have believed for decades that using pot speeds up their reflexes and permits them to produce arpeggios, drum rolls and such that would otherwise be beyond their capacity. In Denmark, however, the Psychochemistry Institute in Copenhagen has taken the trouble to design an objective test and get better information on the question. The study was reported in *Science* (March 2, 1973) by Ole Rafaelsen and his co-workers. "The research design included placebos, a double-blind procedure, tests for reproducibility and dose response, and training effects. . . . The effect of a standard dose of alcohol was also studied."

Using a car simulator, the Danish team gave their subjects varying doses of alcohol and cannabis, the intoxicating element in marijuana. The subjects were tested on their responses to traffic signals and their ability to control the speed of the car and turn the steering wheel.

What the investigators established beyond a reasonable doubt is that, while marijuana does increase the pulse rate and may therefore be considered a stimulant in that respect, in actual driving it increases the time that it takes a user to brake his car in an emergency or to start when the traffic light turns green. It did not induce significant errors in steering, but it definitely reduced the ability of the user to judge the speed of his car and keep it going at a constant speed. In other words, the use of pot while driving is as dangerous as drinking and you'll avoid it if you want to stay alive and whole.

Equally dangerous, peculiarly, are some of the drugs doctors recommend to their patients. Some interesting information about that was reported recently by Dr. Thorne Butler, who analyzes blood samples of drivers suspected by the Las Vegas police of driving under the influence of alcohol. Such a procedure may seem excessively elaborate to you, but it's a great deal more just than relying on the opinion of a policeman. And Dr. Butler says that he finds that about 20 percent of those who are picked up for erratic driving that might indicate drunkenness actually have little or no alcohol in their blood. What do they have? Sedatives and tranquilizers that their doctors have prescribed for their nerves.

Even among the 80 percent who do have appreciable levels of blood alcohol, 16 percent are also sedated by drugs. So be aware that those pills that improve your ability to cope with pressure at the office may be precisely what will render you unable to cope with the emergencies of driving.

As Dr. Butler has said, quoted in *Medical World News* for February 16, 1973, "Our present findings imply that the reality of the drug scene is much greater than a matter of 'pot' and heroin. It involves large numbers of people who are receiving drugs on legitimate prescriptions, and it raises the question: shouldn't physicians instruct patients more carefully about sedatives and warn them about driving?"

An even more unexpected cause of incompetent handling of cars in emergencies has been uncovered by H. J. Roberts, an internist and researcher into traffic accidents. In 1971 he published a book, *The Causes, Ecology and Prevention of Traffic Accidents* (Charles C Thomas, Springfield, Ill.), in which he states that a "significant source" of many unexplained accidents is that "millions of American drivers are subject to pathologic drowsiness and hypoglycemia due to functional hyperinsulinism."

In simpler terms, he is saying that many drivers are susceptible to an abnormal drop in blood sugar which fogs their minds. It isn't that they're starved, but that insulin, which is produced by the pancreas to remove excess sugar from the bloodstream, is being secreted in excessively large quantities. Hence the term "hyperinsulinism." As a result, too much sugar is swept out of the circulating blood and into the body tissues, where it is stored as fat. The trouble comes—and comes fast—when the brain is deprived of its normal supply of glucose circulating in the blood. The brain is extraordinarily sensitive to these levels, and is unable to function properly when the supply is reduced even slightly. Depending on the person and the relative deficiency of glucose in his blood, the result may be anything from an overwhelming sleepiness to a psychotic episode. One of the most common symptoms of a brain deprived of glucose is a kind of stupor, or trancelike state. The automobile driver undergoing such an attack is still able to hold his foot on the gas pedal but may be unaware of what he is doing.

And what is the root cause of this excessive secretion of insulin? Dr. Roberts has no doubts about the answer: "The apparent increased incidence of hyperinsulinism and of narcolepsy [abnormal attacks of sleepiness] during recent decades can be largely attributed to the consequences of an enormous rise in sugar consumption by a vulnerable population."

The basic point Roberts is making is that the human body, and the islets of Langerhans in the pancreas, which secrete insulin, are simply not designed to control efficiently the huge amounts of sugar which modern man consumes. The islets' beta cells become overtaxed and malfunction. Sometimes they produce flawed insulin that is no longer able to remove sugar from the blood—the condition known as maturity-onset diabetes. And sometimes they produce too much insulin and remove too much sugar—hypoglycemia.

But do we really eat that much sugar? Let's look at the facts. According to testimony given to a U.S. Senate panel in February, 1973, by Dr. George M. Briggs, professor of nutrition at the University of California (Berkeley), Americans are eating, on a per capita basis, 102 pounds of table sugar (sucrose) and 14 pounds of corn sugar (dextrose) a year. Consider that fruits contain generous amounts of natural sugar; that vegetable starch and animal protein can be transformed to sugar in the body, and that these values are *in addition* to the 116 pounds of table and corn sugar (the latter being frequently added to processed foods). Consider, too, that the figures for sugar consumption are on a per capita basis, including infants and children, which means that many adults actually eat far more than 116 pounds of refined sugar a year. Millions undoubtedly eat more than their own body weight in sugar every year.

Our rate of sugar consumption is steadily rising, too. At present, it is about twice what it was at the turn of the century. But even that early figure is much more than man ate during the millennia that his physiology evolved and adapted to his eating habits.

To the automobile driver (and the pedestrian!) a sugar-ravaged pancreas may be the prelude to shattered bones and mangled flesh. Let's take a look at what might be a typical example of a driver with an unrecognized tendency toward hyperinsulinism. Jerry wakes up in the morning, takes a cup of coffee with one-and-a-half teaspoons of sugar, and then adds another teaspoon because the Danish he eats with it is so sweet the coffee tastes flat by comparison. Thus fortified with "breakfast," Jerry hops into his car and begins driving to work. Five minutes later, he feels a little groggy, so he lights a cigarette—his third of the day. Once at work, he immediately downs a Coke and lights another cigarette to get another perk-up. Two hours, three cups of coffee, five cigarettes and a candy bar later, Jerry jumps back into his car and goes roaring off to see a customer, but he never gets there. Instead, he winds up at the hospital, where his face is sewn up with twelve stitches. Police tell him he hit his steering wheel after he slammed into the rear of a car stopped for a light. Jerry calls his wife and tells her he's had an "accident." Unfortunately, she believes him. Worse, Jerry believes it himself.

Let's backtrack and see what really caused the "accident." First,

Jerry is one of many people in the United States—Roberts estimates about ten million—who have a tendency toward faulty sugar metabolism. When he woke up in the morning, his blood sugar was somewhat low—which is normal. But what he ate for "breakfast" was abnormal—typical, perhaps, but biochemically grotesque just the same. Into his system first thing in the morning went large amounts of sugar, which to the islets of Langerhans is like reveille played on a klaxon. As if that weren't enough, the sugar was dissolved in coffee. Coffee, of course, contains caffeine. Everyone knows that. What everyone doesn't know is that caffeine increases the level of blood glucose. The nicotine from his cigarettes also caused Jerry's system to raise its glucose level. So much insulin is called out by the hypoglycemic's system that the added glucose, *plus some of the original glucose,* is wiped out in a matter of minutes. Insulin is a firm policeman. In a hypoglycemic such as Jerry, it can be downright brutal.

As his insulin began to vanquish his glucose, Jerry felt tired again. So he drank some Coke, which contains not only large amounts of sugar, but a generous dollop of caffeine as well—ounce for ounce, about one-third as much as coffee. After several hours of assaulting his system with bombardments of sugar, Jerry got behind the wheel of his car. Meanwhile, his hyperinsulinism got behind the wheel of his brain, and began playing games with his entire central nervous system. According to various studies cited by Roberts, it may have disturbed his vision, caused muscle cramps in his arms or legs, made him unusually aggressive, or reduced him to a temporary state of imbecility. In severe cases, the lack of glucose can actually damage nerves by causing water and sodium to migrate into nerve tissue, Roberts states. In Jerry's case, the net result of his sugar-induced hyperinsulinism was that he drove his car into the car in front of his, and Jerry's head went into the steering wheel. An *accident? Appointment* is more like it.

Dr. Roberts estimates that there may be ten million potential Jerrys in the United States.

The threat posed to drivers by hyperinsulinism-induced hypoglycemia can be aggravated by many other factors. One is simply age. Roberts cites a number of studies which show that, on the average, about three out of four "elderly" people have faulty sugar metabolism. Another aggravating factor, Roberts says, is the wide use of such medications as tranquilizers and antihistamines, which have a marked tendency to induce drowsiness. If the user of such drugs is already subject to narcolepsy from hypoglycemia, the combined effect on his behavior behind the wheel can be devastating.

What to do, then, to avoid a possibly fatal collision with hypoglycemia? The obvious answer is to use sugar very sparingly. It wouldn't hurt to eliminate completely all sweets and to stop sugaring your coffee and breakfast cereal. Such a heroic measure is probably not necessary, but a reduction in sugar intake can only benefit anyone's health. Our fathers had the energy to fight the American revolution on a per capita sugar intake of about four pounds a year, and that also gave them the mental energy to write the Declaration of Independence and the Constitution. Your body can get all the glucose it needs from any food you eat. It can even manufacture glucose from the protein in meats. Roberts suggests a diet "that is relatively high in protein, adequate in fat, and devoid of added glucose and sucrose." Even if you don't go quite that far, keep it under control.

You will not be impervious to other dangers, of course, including other drivers with uncontrolled hypoglycemia. But bringing sanity to your metabolism and central nervous system is surely one positive step toward greater safety for you and your family, both on and off the highway.

15 Cadmium, Blood Pressure, and Our Daily Bread

Presumably you are now back to lunching sometimes on tuna salad on toast, since you now know that the tuna will not give you mercury poisoning and will, in fact, protect you against mercury from other sources. A great food, tuna. I wish one could say as much about the toast.

Unfortunately, the white bread from which the toast is made, even if the enriched variety, is as polluted and dangerous a food as one can conceive. Since it is tasteless as well it ought to be easy to give up. But those delicious hot rolls at your favorite restaurant are just as bad and a lot harder to resist. And we are a sandwich-eating country, and how do you make a sandwich without bread?

Yet the simple fact is that American white bread is chockfull of dangerous ingredients, and except for an excessive number of carbohydrate calories, gives you nothing in the way of nutrition. In 1970, Dr. Roger J. Williams, the noted biochemist of the University of Texas at Austin, reported to the National Academy of Science a test with laboratory rats fed the identical "enriched" bread consumed by most Americans. After ninety days, two-thirds of the rats were dead of malnutrition. His statement that "today's bread has about the same nutritional value as sawdust" met with a response from the baking and milling industry that "bread is not customarily consumed alone." Dr. Williams' reply: "Sawdust, when accompanied by good food (milk, meat and cheese) can yield acceptable results, yet sawdust is known to be devoid of nutritional value."

The flour-milling process destroys most of the nutrients of grain. The United States uses the process called "70 percent extraction" whereby 30 percent of the wheat is discarded, including most of the germ and the bran. The bran (containing the first three layers) is first removed. Then follows the aleurone, rich in protein, minerals and useful essential fatty acids. The germ also contains a high percentage of the protein, natural sugars, wheat oil and large amounts of minerals and vitamins. Nearly all the natural valuable nutrients of grains are lost.

Milling also removes 40 percent of the chromium; 50 percent of the pantothenic acid; 30 percent of the choline; 67 percent of the riboflavin; 86 percent of the manganese; 16 percent of the selenium; 78 percent of the zinc; 76 percent of the iron; 89 percent of the cobalt; 60 percent of the calcium; 78 percent of the sodium; 77 percent of the potassium; 85 percent of the magnesium; 71 percent of the phosphorus; 77 percent of the vitamin B_1; 67 percent of the folic acid; most of the vitamin A; 81 percent of the vitamin B_3; 72 percent of the vitamin B_6; most of the vitamin D; and 86 percent of the vitamin E.

These natural elements are essential in our diet. Heart-attack and diabetes victims are deficient in chromium. Depriving experimental animals of chromium tends to cause fatty deposits to build up in the inner walls of their blood vessels. Chickens deprived of manganese grow improperly and become sterile. Liver deterioration results in rats and chickens deprived of selenium. Deficiency of zinc produces high blood pressure, in an indirect way.

Zinc does not seem to have any direct effect on blood pressure, yet it is vital to the maintenance of normal pressure. Why? Because it is one of the very few natural food substances that will detoxify cadmium, an otherwise poisonous metal that is present in food. Cadmium, a heavy metal, is retained in the 70 percent portion of the wheat that goes into flour, while the zinc that could neutralize its harmful effect is milled away.

It is Dr. Henry Schroeder of the Dartmouth Trace Elements Laboratory, who has done the most to uncover the relationship between cadmium, high blood pressure and the steep rate at which Americans are suffering strokes. He was led to investigate the question when Dr. Isabel H. Tipton, a pathologist, found during investigations at the University of Tennessee that victims of cardiovascular disease—especially strokes—also had high levels of the trace element cadmium in their bodies.

Schroeder thought the discovery might be highly significant. But to explore it he had to leave his laboratory in the department of physiology at Dartmouth Medical School. An atmosphere totally free of trace elements was needed. "Environmental conditions in laboratories and animal quarters in most medical schools offered such a spectrum of contaminants that the work we envisioned was not economically possible," Schroeder says. "Nor is it possible in cities without enormous expense, for the air is highly contaminated with metals." The solution was an uncontaminated mountaintop in Vermont. There an animal laboratory was built entirely of wood. All material to be used in the building was analyzed for both lead and cadmium. Mountain spring water was kept pure of trace minerals. Even the air was electrostatically filtered to remove metals. The laboratory itself was almost entirely free of metal objects. No visitors were allowed and even those conducting the experiment were required to remove their shoes before entering the animal quarters.

The rats were divided into several groups of one hundred or more. Then, to the diet of each group small traces of a different single metal were added, and the effects observed. When the additive was cadmium, the results were conclusive. "When the rats were given traces of cadmium in drinking water from the time of weaning, hypertension [high blood pressure] began to appear after about a year of age [increasing the incidence with age]. Once hypertensive, they remained so until death."

Schroeder remarked that the hypertension in rats bore a remarkable similarity to the same disease in human beings. Another observation: sizable plaques were found to form in the aortas [coronary arteries] of mice fed on cadmium. "Hearts were also enlarged," said Schroeder, "renal arteriolar sclerosis [hardening of the kidney artery] was found frequently and some of the systolic blood pressures were over 260 mm Hg." Apparently, the mice were not only suffering high blood pressure because of the cadmium, but were also developing potentially fatal atherosclerosis.

In another experiment, Dr. Schroeder gave cadmium to a group of rats from the time they were weaned. Within thirteen months, nine of the twenty-two rats developed hypertension.

Then the researcher decided to remove the cadmium from the livers of these rodents. He used a special chemical capable of binding with cadmium to remove it from the system. One week after a single injection, the hypertensive rats became normal and their blood pressure fell from 169 to an average of 82.8. With cadmium removed the zinc levels rose. Even though the rats were put back on their cadmium diets, their blood pressures remained normal for about two months.

"Therefore," said Schroeder, "we established that rats fed or injected with small doses of cadmium became hypertensive, that removal of some of the cadmium results in a return to normo-tension, and that a high ratio of renal cadmium to zinc is usually associated with hypertension."

To this day, Dr. Schroeder is not sure of the precise relationship between cadmium and zinc. One of Schroeder's colleagues, Dr. Douglas Frost, explains that zinc is a natural metabolic antagonist of cadmium. The liver and kidneys, and to a lesser extent other body tissues, store both cadmium and zinc. "The body has problems differentiating between cadmium and zinc," said Dr. Frost.

"Apparently it may store cadmium instead of zinc under some circumstances."

If there is a deficit of zinc in the diet, the body may make this deficit up by storing cadmium instead, it appears. On the other hand, if dietary zinc intake is kept high, zinc will be stored and cadmium will be excreted. That appears the most likely explanation for the results Schroeder observed with his laboratory rats. And Schroeder has been successful in reversing hypertension in the rodents by replacing the cadmium with zinc.

Can these findings have any significance for human beings?

When excessively high levels of minerals accumulate in the body, the urine will contain large amounts of them. The rule holds true for cadmium. Researchers have reported that the urine of hypertensive patients contained up to forty times as much cadmium as did the urine of normotensive persons. If this isn't proof that cadmium levels and hypertension are related, it is at least strong evidence.

There's a good chance, in fact, that what doctors now consider normal blood pressure is really not normal at all, but abnormally high. That would be one explanation for the fact that Americans have both higher "normal" blood pressure and higher cadmium levels than a good many other people of the world.

Where do we get all that cadmium from? Dozens of places. Some of it floats around in the air, emitted from smokestacks as a by-product of commercial zinc and copper production. Some water supplies contain large amounts of the trace mineral. Most of it, however, comes from the foods we eat and the beverages we drink. Phosphate fertilizers contain five to ten parts per million of cadmium. That's a significant amount when you're talking about trace minerals. A number of plants absorb the cadmium from fertilizers and pass it on to your dinner table.

"The practice of refining wheat and polishing rice has interesting effects on the relative amounts of cadmium and zinc contained in the finished grain," says Schroeder. "Cadmium is distributed throughout the endosperm and germ; zinc is concentrated in the germ and bran. Refined white flour contains only six to nine per cent of the zinc in the whole grain, all of it bound to gluten, but the cadmium content rises with refining. . . .

"This practice leads to a disturbed ratio of cadmium to zinc ingested of 1:17, compared to 1:120 in whole wheat."

Schroeder also warns, "Areas of the world where the major source of calories comes from refined grains are apt to show a high incidence of hypertension, although tea, coffee and seafood may also contribute much cadmium."

Schroeder's reference to tea and coffee is not a casual one. He says that a liter—above five cups—of coffee or tea a day actually *doubles* the average daily intake of cadmium! That factor in itself could go a long way toward explaining why cadmium levels are so high in this country.

Softness of the drinking water, which makes the water low in zinc as in other minerals, plays a part in hypertension, too, according to Schroeder. In another experiment in his laboratory, the researcher put some rats on a cadmium-rich diet. Within five hundred days, a full 80 percent of the animals that were fed soft water had developed hypertension. Only 17.7 percent of those on hard water developed the disease. Autopsies later showed that the cadmium-zinc ratios were about 1.0 for the rats on soft water. The normal rats had ratios of less than 0.5.

Yet suppose you live in New York City or Boston, where the drinking water is soft. How are you going to avoid it? How many people are going to give up coffee because it has a dangerously high content of cadmium? If we were the kind of people who could stop drinking the coffee we love and switch to 100 percent whole-wheat bread, even though we don't care for its taste, we would be a different breed of animal. We wouldn't have to worry about pollution because we would just make the sacrifices necessary to eliminate it.

As you and I know, people can give up a favorite food if it

makes them sick within twenty-four hours. But what about giving up something they are told will hurt them in ten or thirty years? Not likely.

It is obviously more productive to look for ways to counteract the cadmium we are receiving, the first and most obvious of which is to increase the zinc in our diets. It takes a little doing, however, since the nature of our food is such that actually millions of us are deficient in zinc.

According to a paper presented by Dr. Walter J. Pories of the University of Rochester School of Medicine and Dentistry at the American Association for the Advancement of Science meetings in 1968, right now the soils of thirty-two different states in the United States are deficient in zinc. There are several reasons for this. Zinc is naturally low in leached-out soils such as those found in many coastal areas. It is also made unavailable by chelation in alkaline soils, in those very high in carbon compounds, and where there are high concentrations of magnesium or phosphate—frequently found in clay soils. And, Pories adds, "More recently, heavy fertilization of soils with phosphates and nitrogens have contributed greatly to zinc deficiency of soils and thus of crops."

In Grandma's day, the problem was not so critical. Although the mineral was probably deficient in the American food, we received great quantities of it from artificial sources in our environment. Galvanized pipes, pots and pans were a constant supply of zinc. But recently we have been getting away from galvanized items.

Yet, even as the zinc in our diets dwindles, research is showing that, in addition to counteracting cadmium, we need zinc for a good many reasons. According to Dr. Pories, zinc is now recognized by researchers as an essential element for all animals including man. It is required in only minute concentrations—from 20 to 100 parts per million—"yet even slight or moderate deficiencies can retard growth, lower feed efficiency, and inhibit general well being."

About fifteen years ago researchers learned that dietary zinc deficiency caused animals to develop ulcers and scaling skin. Minor wounds failed to heal, disorders developed in bones and joints, there was a severe decline in fertility. Yet, ironically, more than five years passed before researchers realized that man, too, needed zinc and could suffer from a deficiency of the mineral.

One of the most important recent medical findings is that zinc plays a big role in the healing of wounds. Even in ancient Egypt, zinc was applied topically to wounds in the form of calamine. But it wasn't until the 1950s that "modern" medicine gave the mineral proper attention in this important area. It was Dr. Pories who made the original discovery—by accident. "We were studying wound healing in rats and trying to control the rate of repair by addition of various amino acid analogs to the diet." One of the ingredients added was beta-phenyllactic acid, a chemical expected to retard healing. "To our surprise," reports Pories, "it definitely accelerated healing. We repeated the work several times and in every instance healing was promoted."

Upon further investigation, Pories discovered that it was not beta-phenyllactic acid which caused the healing, but a chemical used in its manufacture—zinc. "A series of 10 subsequent experiments proved that zinc was the beneficial contaminant," the doctor says. In those experiments, wounds healed up to 40 percent faster in old male rats, and up to 20 percent faster in young males and old females.

In 1965, Pories decided to test his findings on human beings. He selected twenty young airmen suffering from a condition which caused hair to grow in the sinuses, resulting in infection and pus. Each of the men underwent surgery. Afterward, ten of the patients were placed on 220 milligrams of zinc sulfate three times daily. The other ten were given their usual diets without the supplementation.

"The difference was dramatic. Although the medicated patients had larger wounds than the controls, the airmen treated with the zinc healed 34.3 days faster. This study demonstrated that zinc plays a role in human healing and the administration of this element can benefit healing in humans." These results are not unique. Pories presented numerous cases in which the results were equally glowing. He also made it clear that zinc deficiency in hospital patients admitted because of wounds or undergoing surgery prolongs their stay unduly.

If we could eat plenty of clams and oysters, none of us would ever have to worry about too little zinc. Shellfish accumulate the mineral in large quantities. But it does seem foolish to risk hepatitis in order to avoid high blood pressure. Zinc-rich foods you can eat safely include ocean fish, nuts and seeds. Although they all possess other virtues, just their rich stores of zinc can vastly benefit you if you eat enough of them. Wheat germ is an excellent zinc-rich food that can be included in your daily diet with little trouble or expense. You can eat it for breakfast, like President Nixon. You can sprinkle it on salads, add some to stewed tomatoes, hamburger or casserole dishes.

But when you're all through, though you will surely have benefited, you still will have no way of knowing you have eaten enough zinc to counteract all the cadmium this polluted world is putting into you. For cadmium is also polluting the air wherever there are cars. You are almost certain to be exposed to it any time you go near a street or highway. Ralph Nader's Center for the Study of Responsive Law has warned that an undetermined number of gasoline brands contain cadmium (February 12, 1971). The toxic metal has also been found in tires, as well as heating and lubricating oils. As an air pollutant, cadmium gets into water supplies and food plants, especially cereal grains. Cadmium pollution is growing in intensity and thus is probably too extensive to be countered by zinc-rich foods alone.

Happily it has been established that vitamin C is a good protector against cadmium specifically. The latest report on the effectiveness of ascorbic acid to detoxify and render harmless the cadmium in the environment appeared in *Science* (September 4, 1970). M. R. Spivey Fox and Bert E. Fry, Jr., two scientists in the Food and Drug Administration's Division of Nutrition, added cadmium to the diet of young Japanese quail. They selected this bird because of its exceptionally rapid growth rate and extreme sensitivity to dietary deficits and toxic materials. The Japanese quail is far more sensitive to pollution than human beings, and anything found to aid the survival of this delicate bird would almost certainly be of even greater value to people.

Day-old birds of both sexes were placed on an adequate diet of purified soybean protein. Some birds ate the food alone; others ate food plus cadmium (seventy-five milligrams per kilogram of feed) or ascorbic acid (vitamin C) in varying doses; still others ate food plus a combination of cadmium and vitamin C. After four weeks of testing, the birds were weighed. These results alone showed that young birds fed cadmium failed to gain weight as rapidly as the other birds. In fact, seven of the fifty-one birds which ate cadmium died, while all twenty-four on the cadmium-free regimen survived. However, the depressed growth rate was corrected by the addition of vitamin C to the diet. In this experiment the blood of the quails was sampled and their livers were removed, weighed and assayed for zinc, iron, copper and cadmium content. While the cadmium concentration was high in all birds receiving the metal, whether or not they got vitamin C, other measurements showed a startling protective effect from the cadmium by vitamin C.

Without exception, every bird exposed to cadmium developed anemia. Liver stores of iron were sharply depleted by the toxic metal. But that's half the story; the other half is that even the smallest supplement of dietary ascorbic acid brought significant improvement in the birds' ability to use the iron in their bodies, even though the amounts used were not enough to correct the anemia completely.

It would seem clear from the study of Fox and Fry that once

again vitamin C has proven its value as a protector against a host of toxic materials—in this case cadmium. Make sure you get plenty of it, plus zinc-rich foods, and you should be well protected against this particular pollutant of our food, our air and our water.   There is still a third protector, however—our old friend sodium alginate. By this time you should be including it in your prepared foods for protection against lead and strontium 90. It also handles cadmium in the same way. It chelates whatever cadmium it meets in the gut and carries it out of the body. So please don't forget to use sodium alginate in your cooking. It's one of the best aids you have.

16 Germs That Protect Your Gut

Whether you know it or not—and you probably don't—we have all had salmonella poisoning. Not that it is possible to have this wretched bacterial infection without being aware of it. You get intestinal cramps and severe diarrhea. You may vomit repeatedly. You run a fever and you feel utterly miserable.

Naturally, you call the doctor. He may come and see you. More likely, though, he makes a quick, incisive, positive—and wrong—diagnosis over the telephone. Intestinal flu, summer flu, the twenty-four-hour virus, virus X—these are all devious ways of saying that your doctor doesn't know what's wrong with you and isn't even going to try to find out because he knows from experience that it's going to pass in three days at most. So he calls the drugstore and sends you a tranquilizer that stops the vomiting and puts you to sleep. In a couple of days you get better, and modern scientific medicine has triumphed once again.

Salmonellosis is everywhere. A bacterial infection that is a milder first cousin of typhoid fever, it is diagnosable only by laboratory tests that take at least twenty-four hours to complete. By the time a sample is sent to the lab for testing and reported, the attack is passing and it's too late to treat it. So you really can't blame your doctor for not bothering.

And as a consequence, although the communicable-disease section of the U.S. Public Health Service estimates that there are at least three million cases a year of salmonella poisoning, and maybe two or three times as many, the annual reported cases run only into the thousands. All the rest are accepted as "virus."

Salmonella poisoning is our most widespread unrecognized disease, reaching epidemic proportions every summer. People commonly get it from eggs and egg products such as mayonnaise, baked goods and premium ice cream. The infectious organism is common in meat, is surprisingly frequent in dried coconut flakes, and is commonly found in almost any type of food that is improperly stored in a freezer. In the summer of 1963 in the northeastern section of the United States, serious outbreaks of this form of food poisoning swept through forty hospitals, sickening many and leaving sixteen known dead. All through the summer months, when the salmonella bacteria grow best, new highs for incidence of the disease were reported.

The Public Health Service galloped in, and traced the outbreaks in Philadelphia hospitals to Grade-B eggs from a farm near that city. Hospitals often purchase grade-B eggs, which may be cracked, to save money. In this case, the cost cutting turned out to be very costly indeed.

Poisoning from the various strains of this intestinal bacteria reached epidemic proportions in the middle of the summer. The PHS reported that 775 cases of sickness from *Salmonella derby* alone were recorded by July 17, and that about 20 cases a week were noted after that. A warning was issued cautioning citizens to cook all their eggs thoroughly and to avoid eating cracked eggs.

Such salmonella types as *derby, typhimurium,* and *thompson* may invade the cracked eggs and pass through the membrane surrounding the egg contents. A human being, or almost any mammal, who eats a contaminated egg is in for a lot of trouble, unless he has the friendly intestinal flora that provide natural protection.

Cooking will usually destroy the disease organism, but few of the cases were from home-cooked eggs. The average housewife buys grade-A eggs, which are clean and free from cracks. Most of the danger lies in the bulk eggs used by institutions, commercial bakeries or restaurants. Procedures and sanitation are often lax, and the salmonella germ has a good chance to spread.

There are plants which sell the bulk eggs, but health officials found little danger there. The eggs are shipped to the plants in cold storage. Egg-cracking machines automatically separate the whites from the yolks, and the separate liquids are poured into cartons. They are then flash-frozen at thirty degrees below zero and shipped frozen to bakeries or restaurants. Bakeries leave the huge cans of eggs standing open on counters to thaw, and might not use all the eggs for several days. This practice invites the invasion and growth of disease organisms such as salmonella.

It is one way large-scale food processing sometimes creates unnecessary health threats. The individual can examine his eggs for defects, but with modern "convenience foods," you must take what you get. The egg is one of nature's best foods, filled with minerals and vitamins. Like all highly nutritious foods, it is highly susceptible to contamination. When allowed to thaw after freezing and stand exposed in a warm bakery or restaurant, it will turn bad. Cooking is relied on to kill the deadly bacteria again, but judging by the growing epidemics of food poisoning, it is not as reliable as the industry apologists like to think it is.

Frozen bulk eggs are also used in the food industry wherever great batches are called for, as in commercial cake mixes or powdered eggs. These products have been most troublesome sources of salmonella poisoning. Some egg products made in the United State are exported, causing food poisoning in the countries of destination.

The problem in Great Britain with imported salmonella was quickly realized, and appropriate steps were taken to counteract it. No liquid or frozen whole egg, whether home-grown or imported, may be used in the preparation of food for human consumption in Britain unless it has been pasteurized. The *British Medical Journal* (September 28, 1963), commenting on the law, said,

This important commodity [frozen eggs], through its widespread use in food-manufacturing establishments, including bakeries and hospitals, has for many years been responsible for outbreaks of . . . food poisoning infections with salmonella *typhimurium, salmonella thompson,* and other salmonella serotypes. Everyone who has the health of his country at heart will welcome the introduction of regulations designed to render the product safe.

. . . It was clear from the epidemiological pattern of the outbreaks that repetition of similar incidents could be treated only by treating bulked egg material at the production stage. The hygiene of poultry husbandry, of the egg cracking stations, and of the bakery could not hope to control the spread of contamination by infected egg.

What is being done in the United States, where the salmonella problem is even more serious? The Food and Drug Administration has not put forth any regulatory plan for pasteurizing bulked egg because it says pasteurizing would change the consistency of the egg white. It has announced that the poultry industry is working on the problem, and FDA scientists are spot-checking occasional batches of eggs, an obviously futile approach.

The American Public Health Association has been threatening to sue the Department of Agriculture because the department's labels are deceiving the American housewife. For years, the American housewife has been lulled into a false sense of security by such phrases as "U.S. Inspected" and "U.S. Inspected for Wholesomeness" on meat and poultry packages, says the A.P.H.A. These labels imply a degree of purity that is not necessarily there, because federal meat inspectors do not check for salmonella and other common food-poisoning bacteria. Thus, unless a housewife handles meat or poultry with care, it can bring the whole family down with a devastating case of salmonellosis.

Dr. Oscar J. Sussman, president of the New Jersey Public Health Association and head of the national association's task force which is considering legal action against the government, said several studies have identified salmonella as a consistent contaminant in meat (Washington *Post,* November 8, 1971). Although the 1967 Wholesome Meat Act and the 1968 Wholesome Poultry Products Act prohibit using the government seal of approval on any raw meat or poultry which is adulterated, unwholesome and in any way injurious to health, misbranded or improperly labeled and provide that "the public will be informed of the manner of handling required to maintain the article in wholesome condition," recent studies indicate that many pieces of government-inspected poultry and meat may be contaminated with salmonella. The bacteria are killed by thorough cooking. But, warns Sussman, consumers can contaminate utensils and other foods unless they wash their hands after handling the contaminated foods.

Certainly the housewife should be careful about washing her hands after handling meat, and about keeping one cutting board strictly reserved for meat and not using it for cutting vegetables, fruits or bread. These precautions might reduce the incidence of food poisoning. But the real problem goes much deeper. The question public-health officials should be posing is, "Why is so much of our meat and poultry contaminated with salmonella in the first place?"

A major part of the problem is related to the widespread use of antibiotics in animal feeds, says Dr. David H. Smith in the *New England Journal of Medicine* (September 22, 1966). These antibiotics are used not to improve the health of the animal or the consumer, but to fatten up the animal so that this increased weight will bring the cattle breeder more profit.

Dr. Herbert S. Goldberg, professor of microbiology at the University of Missouri School of Medicine, told a Food and Drug Law Institute symposium in Washington, D.C., in the summer of 1966 that more than half of the $114,600,000 worth of antibiotics sold each year in the United States—1,800,000 pounds—were used in animal feeds or added to food crops.

Dairy cows are fed the drugs along with their ordinary feed. So the United States Department of Agriculture and the Food and Drug Administration are kept continually busy seizing shipments of milk contaminated with antibiotics.

According to the World Health Organization booklet *The Public Health Aspects of the Use of Antibiotics in Food and Feedstuffs,* published in 1963, some apple and pear orchards are now being treated with strepto-antibiotics in an attempt to fight fruit diseases. So are beans, celery, cucumber, hops, peppers, lettuce, potatoes, sesame, tomatoes, walnuts and cherries.

According to the same report, antibiotics are now used to preserve fish and poultry. Chickens are dipped in antibiotic solutions after slaughter. Fish may also be thrown into a tub of antibiotic solution as soon as they are caught, or the fillets may be washed with the drug.

Steers are sometimes injected with antibiotics just before they are slaughtered as a means of preserving the meat.

All this is bad news, indeed.

In 1960 the Council on Foods and Nutrition of the American Medical Association published a report in the AMA *Journal* (June 4, 1960) stating, "Under proper conditions, certain antibiotics are desirable, useful additives for extending the market life of some foods." Yet, even then, the AMA inadvertently touched upon what has grown to be an incredibly serious health problem. "Development of resistant forms of organisms under intended conditions of use presents a serious problem," the report went on. And that's about all the AMA had to say.

Seven years later, in the October 5, 1967, issue of *The New Scientist* the problem was stated a bit more emphatically:

Antibiotics on the Farm—Major Threat to Human Health.

There is now a mass of evidence showing that the misuse of antibiotics as growth-promoting food supplements and as mass prophylactic agents has caused a serious increase in bacterial drug resistance in recent years. The threat to human and animal health has been made abundantly clear, and warnings from experts in the field have mounted over the past year.

Why precisely is this ceaseless bombardment with antibiotics harmful to us?

Antibiotics in animal feed and dips before freezing are usually very effective against the salmonella bacteria, which cause salmonellosis. That means that they are successful in destroying almost all of the salmonella. Yet even the most powerful antibiotics never destroy absolutely all of the disease-causing organisms. A few of the bacteria are hardy enough to survive. Later, when they reproduce, the new bacteria tend to inherit the qualities which make them tough enough to survive attacks by the antibiotic. Those new bacteria develop what the medical profession calls "drug resistance." What it means to you and me is that, the next time we contract salmonellosis, it will not be as easily treated with antibiotics.

As a matter of fact, precisely this problem has occurred in treating salmonellosis in Great Britain, according to *The New Scientist*. And there is little or no doubt that, as antibiotic resistance increases year by year, so does the likelihood that any given animal carcass will be infected with salmonella—for which food inspectors do not inspect. And, according to Dr. W. E. C. Moore of the Veterinary Science Department of Virginia's Polytechnic Institute, it is the antibiotics in poultry feed that lead directly to salmonella contamination of eggs, chicken and turkey.

On March 26, 1971, the FDA said that it had found samples from 100,000 cartons of a whipping cream, which had already been distributed under twenty-five different brand names, to be contaminated with salmonella bacteria. Less than a month later, the FDA revealed the recall of 1,848 boxes of egg noodles contaminated with salmonella. Stores in Minnesota, Wisconsin and the Dakotas were told to return their shipments. Such discoveries, of course, are only a drop in the bucket. Most of the contaminated food gets through to the consumer, who in many cases further breeds the contamination himself.

When you buy, say, frozen breaded shrimp, the breading may contain so few viable salmonella organisms that, even if the food were inspected, it would pass. The cold of the market freezer, which is kept at zero degrees, prevents them from increasing. But in your home freezer the temperature may be fifteen or twenty degrees, which permits the organisms to multiply. When you thaw the food, the bacteria multiply rapidly. Then, if you refreeze it, they go on multiplying, and by the time you get to eating it, there are billions of the bacteria in the food.

They will be destroyed if the food is cooked thoroughly so that the innermost portion is heated to 160 degrees. But, when it's a convenience food that is merely warmed and served, it frequently is just not warmed enough. You know what the result of that is.

You may as well take it for granted. You can hardly hope to escape eating food contaminated with salmonella.

But you can protect yourself.

It was discovered recently in an encouraging experiment with two mouse colonies that natural whole food gives you an added bonus—a precious substance called pacifarins, which, it was shown in a most unusual experiment, confers a natural immunity to salmonellosis.

Dr. Howard A. Schneider of the Institute for Biomedical Research of the American Medical Association found that the outer portion of wheat, corn, rye and rice—the part that is discarded when the grain is refined—provides some factor akin to an antibiotic which can prevent salmonella infections in laboratory mice. His experiments are described in *Science* (November 3, 1967).

When Dr. Schneider and his colleagues fed two mouse colonies different diets and then infected both with salmonella, one group had a notably higher survival rate. Ninety out of one hundred lived; in the other group, ninety out of a hundred died. The group with the high fatalities were fed a precisely assembled semi-synthetic diet containing all the known required amino acids (protein), carbohydrates, vitamins and minerals, a diet which was perhaps more complete and no more synthetic than that consumed daily by the vast majority of supermarket patrons. The other colony, the one in which ninety out of a hundred lived, was fed a natural diet only. Whole wheat was an important part in the natural diet because of the newly discovered "resistance" factor, pacifarins.

What is the resistance factor? Dr. Schneider never found out. Just as he was really getting his experiments under way, the AMA decided to discontinue its Institute for Biomedical Research.

The best guess Dr. Schneider could make about pacifarins is that they are a kind of antibiotic produced by bacteria that live on the outer husks of grains. Although the odds are in its favor, that guess may or may not be correct. But what does seem beyond dispute is that by eating whole wheat, including the bran, by eating wild rice which comes in the hull, by eating brown rice, whole grain buckwheat and corn on the cob, we can give ourselves an enormous degree of protection against the salmonella bacteria that get into our digestive systems.

It's not easy to buy foods made of such completely unprocessed grains. But you can buy wheat in the hull and cook it up to make a breakfast cereal that tastes better than what you're eating now. You can also use it as a substitute for potatoes at any meal, or stuff a fowl with it.

Whole, unmilled buckwheat is more readily available. It's known as kasha, and simply boiled and served with some gravy, it's delicious. It also goes well as a turkey stuffing, and since frozen turkeys are a frequent source of salmonella infection, it's a very good idea to have the antidote in the stuffing.

Does it seem strange that one type of bacteria should produce the pacifarins that will kill or inhibit another type, salmonella? It shouldn't. There is the same continual warfare raging among germs as among animals in the jungle or people at the pinnacle of civilization. Within our bodies, different kinds of bacteria hold each other in check so that no one becomes dominant.

If one inimical type does gain the upper hand, the result is bacterial infection. We have other defenses against such infections, of course, but most of the time we don't have to use them, because even though there are some infective bacteria like salmonella in our bodies all the time, other harmless germs war against them and keep their numbers from getting too great.

Of these friendly germs, the most important seem to be the lactobacilli—germs that thrive in dairy products and turn them sour by forming lactic acid. We kill them by pasteurization to preserve milk, yet the lactobacilli are of enormous value to our health.

The relationship between salmonella and the power of the acidophilus strain of lactobacilli to destroy it has been noted by visitors to the Near East, according to Arthur and Charles Bryan of Jacksonville University. They recorded their views in an article entitled "Nature's Gastro-intestinal Antibiotics," printed in *Drug and Cosmetic Industry* (March, 1959): "In the near-East, despite the high incidence of . . . salmonella dysenteries among visitors, the natives appear to be comparatively free from these diseases . . . it is noted that daily these near-East peoples consume leben, a composite of thickened salted curds cultured with L. acidophilus."

We all notice headlines in the newspaper periodically reporting outbreaks of food poisoning traceable to salmonella. Sometimes hundreds of people are simultaneously hospitalized after large social functions at which contaminated food was served. Yet there are always a few people who are not affected. The most likely reason is that they are protected by a thriving intestinal fauna.

Lactobacilli in the gut protect us against a variety of infections by holding down the size of the colonies of infectious germs. If you are a woman subject to either of two common vaginal infections, trichomoniasis or candida albicans, you can improve the situation by getting more lactobacilli in your diet. The same bacteria control staph infections and others. And, most importantly, they can make the difference between coming down with salmonellosis and never noticing that you ate contaminated food.

You put them in your gut with the right milk products. Certified raw milk, if you can get it, is an excellent source. (The lactobacilli have been killed in pasteurized milk.) Yogurt is good, but you have to eat it frequently. The Bulgaricus strain of lactobacillus used to make yogurt will survive for only about three days in the human gut. The same is true of buttermilk. But if every day you have either a portion of yogurt, or some sour cream, or a glass of buttermilk, you will be well protected.

You can also easily get a yogurt starter that is the acidophilus strain, and make your own yogurt at home. It's very easy and the directions are right on the package. That will permanently provide you with lactobacilli in your gut, unless you are treated with antibiotics for some reason. The lactobacilli will not overflourish, since an excess simply passes into the stools, where it provides soft bulk that eliminates constipation and reduces unpleasant odors.

There is nothing to fear in putting these living germs into your digestive tract. They are friends and allies, eager to man the outposts salmonella is trying to invade.

17 Polluted Food and a Woman's Breasts

I'd like you to pay some attention to an area of food pollution where there is no hard evidence to prove the danger. On the other hand, neither is there any evidence of safety. I may be wrong and if I'm ever proven so I'll cheerfully admit it and be one happy fellow. Right now I suspect that I'm right, and I'm worried. I think you should be too—particularly if you're a woman.

While some other forms of cancer are decreasing, breast cancer, like lung cancer, keeps increasing. Fortunately, it is often detected in time for a clean cure by removal of one or both breasts. Regardless of the effectiveness of surgical intervention, however, I'm sure you'd rather avoid it. Can it be done?

The causes of breast cancer are unknown, according to medical orthodoxy. But there are some pretty good clues, and they all point to an excess in a woman's system of the female hormone estrogen, particularly its synthetic form, diethylstilbestrol, commonly known as DES. DES, like most carcinogens, acts very slowly and is therefore hard to incriminate beyond a doubt. But about twenty years ago it was a medical fashion to give DES to pregnant women who were threatened with miscarriage on the chance that an insufficient supply of estrogen might have been causing the trouble. In 1972 the effects began showing up in reports that the daughters of such women were beginning to develop vaginal cancers.

The connection with food supply is that for many years DES has been used to speed up the growth of beef cattle. It's not that the cancer-causing potential of the hormone was unknown. By some inexplicable error of judgment, though, it was assumed that if a steer was fed no DES during the last forty-eight hours of its life the hormone would be completely eliminated from the flesh, with no residues.

After many years of protest by assorted consumer advocates, more thorough inspections were instituted. In October, 1971, the Agriculture Department finally confessed to an "inexcusable" error in its claim that no DES residue could be found in beef from cattle that had eaten feed containing DES. At that same time, the FDA admitted that new and better testing procedures have indeed confirmed the presence of DES in the livers of slaughtered animals. In fact, it was found that about one-half of one percent of all beef livers tested showed detectable levels of the hormone. And, since the nation's annual beef slaughter is about 40 million animals, the random-sample analysis would indicate that up to 200,000 slaughtered beef cattle during the year 1971 contained residues of the powerful synthetic hormone.

Having made this incriminating confession, did the government outlaw the use of this hormone, which represents an obvious threat to the health of the consumer? You can bet your pharmaceutical stock it didn't.

Stilbestrol is a powerful stimulant to cattle growth. USDA officials say that just sixteen cents' worth of the hormone produces a weight gain worth about twelve dollars at the slaughterhouse. So the Department of Agriculture continued to insist on the need to allow cattle and sheep raisers to use DES in feed, even though twenty-one other nations have banned it and even though the department itself long ago banned the hormone from chicken feed.

Instead, the FDA made a new regulation. They told cattlemen

to stop using feed containing DES seven days before slaughter—as against forty-eight hours in the old regulations—and to provide certification to this effect. But follow-up inspections found even more DES residues in the animals after the seven-day withdrawal period than had previously been discovered, perhaps because the inspections were more careful. Because the law requires that there must be no detectable residue of any cancer-causing substance in human food, the FDA rather reluctantly was compelled to ban the use of DES in cattle feed, as of January 1, 1973. It offered an alternative, however. Cattle growers are now permitted to implant pellets of the hormone in the ears of their animals, where the pellets slowly dissolve, releasing the hormone into the steers' bloodstreams.

The FDA believes the pellets will leave no residues. It would be nice if they were right, but there is no proof that they are. The evidence would seem to indicate that DES is highly persistent stuff, and that once it gets into an animal's body, it's hard to get it out again.

And that, presumably, goes for us too. So that if we eat a trace of DES in our steak or pot roast or liver three or four times a week, over a period of twenty years it could accumulate into quite a quantity of surplus estrogen, and that, according to strong indications, could induce breast cancer in susceptible women.

One alarming indication is to be found in the work of Dr. Otto Sartorius, director of the Cancer Control Clinic of Santa Barbara General Hospital in California. Dr. Sartorius has found that the DES in birth-control pills causes, at the least, precancerous changes in women's breasts. And, while the quantities of DES involved are far larger than you will ever get from eating meat for a week or a month, they are not so different from the accumulation of many years.

"Women who use the Pill are sustaining irreversible and permanent breast changes. The cancer-risk factor in women taking the Pill is 2.8 times greater the world around than in women who do not use the Pill," Dr. Otto Sartorius stated in an interview with *Prevention* magazine.

Medical articles have reported that "abnormal changes" stop when women stop using the Pill. This is absolutely untrue, Dr. Sartorius emphasized. Present studies indicate that the hormone swallowed today is adversely affecting the breast for the future.

At Santa Barbara General Hospital, Dr. Sartorius examined three thousand patients over a period of three years. He was distressed with the abnormal findings in the breasts of those women who were on the Pill or who *had been* on the Pill. He was amazed to find that, regardless of whether a woman had just started to use the Pill or whether she had been off it for two or three years, her breasts were *harder and more nodular* than those of the women who had never been on the Pill. The changes were so marked they could be discovered just by touch.

In order to confirm this startling finding, Dr. Sartorius did a controlled study on two hundred girls, half of whom had been on the Pill. All the data were collected by his technicians in advance. When he palpated the breasts of each patient, he did not know to which group she belonged. His findings were then compared with the records of his technicians. Just by palpation, Dr. Sartorius had achieved 92 percent accuracy. His results are a very good indicator of just how widespread and profound are changes in the breasts of those using the Pill.

The 1972 Annual Report of the American Cancer Society states that there are 74,000 new cases of breast cancer each year, and 33,000 deaths of this disease. In fact, breast cancer is the leading cause of death by cancer.

"If I were a girl," Dr. Sartorius says, "I would not be on the Pill. The Pill is producing abnormal changes in the breast and I know I wouldn't want them in my breast. What will happen to millions of women with these breast changes? I worry about this."

Most of the pills have a high estrogen level which increases the growth rate of many cancers and also produces the abnormalities that Dr. Sartorius now sees in the breast. "Estrogen is the fodder on which carcinoma grows," he states. "To produce cancer in lower animals, you first introduce an estrogen base."

Presumably the same goes for human beings.

Yet not every woman who uses birth-control pills is going to get cancer, and neither is every woman who eats meat containing DES. Most women, in fact, never will. There must be some other element that comes into play.

There is, says a Philadelphia researcher who has found reason to believe that a woman's ability to fight off a carcinogen like DES and resist the development of breast cancer depends on how much iodine she has in her system.

The researcher is Dr. Bernard A. Eskin, director of endocrinology in the Department of Obstetrics and Gynecology at the Medical College of Pennsylvania. His belief that iodine deficiency may contribute to the development of breast cancer is based on extensive tests of laboratory animals and the beginning of clinical studies with human beings.

Most convincing of all is the fact that his laboratory experiments, showing the effect of iodine deficiency in the development of tumors and other disorders in rat breasts, jibe with known facts about the incidence of human breast cancer in regions of the world that are iodine-deficient. These iodine-poor areas are well plotted in every country—in fact, probably no other single nutrient has been pinpointed around the globe as comprehensively as this one. That is because lack of iodine causes the extremely visible deficiency disease goiter. Iodine is needed by the thyroid gland, located in the throat, to manufacture the hormone thyroxine. In the absence of iodine, the thyroid swells to gross proportions (goiter).

Regions of endemic goiter—that is, areas where goiter is prevalent because iodine is lacking in the soil and food—have been identified for many years. And now, comparing these regions with areas high in breast-cancer deaths, it turns out that the two coincide to a remarkable degree.

Japan and Iceland, for example, have few instances of goiter and few instances of breast cancer. (Japan, where iodine-rich seaweed is a favorite food, has a death rate from breast cancer five times lower than that of the United States.) On the other hand, Mexico and Thailand are high in both goiter and breast cancer. Since these are both countries where babies are commonly breast fed, this information tends to contradict the belief that nursing improves resistance to this form of cancer, while it reinforces the idea that iodine in the diet is a determining factor. Breast-cancer death rates are also high in endemic goiter areas in Poland, Switzerland, Australia, the Soviet Union and the United States. In the United States, the highest death rate from breast cancer anywhere in the country is found in what is known as the "goiter belt" in the Great Lakes region.

"The similarity of high mortality regions to endemic goiter areas is striking," Dr. Eskin told the National Medical Association at its 1971 convention in Philadelphia, where he spoke on his research findings. A lengthy summary of his work over the past few years was earlier published in *Transactions of the New York Academy of Sciences* (December, 1970).

Dr. Eskin's laboratory studies of the effect of iodine levels on tumor development cover a long series of tests done with thousands of laboratory animals. Perhaps the most striking of these is one in which a cancer-causing agent—DMBA—was injected into two hundred rats. Some of the experimental animals had been fed an adequate diet, sufficient in iodine. Others had been made iodine-deficient. While all the animals eventually developed breast tumors from this powerful carcinogen, those that were not protected by iodine did so measurably sooner. In fact, the process of cancer development was speeded up 25 percent in the animals on the iodine-deficient diet.

The protective role of iodine seems to be related in a curious way to the carcinogenic properties of the female sex hormone estrogen. The hormone, which females require for the reproductive process, is naturally produced under delicate controls that normally prevent an excess. There is little reason for a woman to fear her own estrogen production, unless it should get out of control. Similarly, estrogen replacement therapy at menopause, which simply restores normal estrogen levels, is not known to be dangerous. It is the surplus over a woman's normal production, coming from food and contraceptive pills, that is believed to involve danger—particularly if the woman's system contains insufficient iodine. Much of Dr. Eskin's work explores this relationship. It is one of extreme importance to women today, as the investigator stresses.

Dr. Eskin's studies show how the harmful effect of estrogen can be stepped up by iodine deficiency. As has long been known, estrogen causes breast cancer in several animal species—in fact, estrogen administration is a standard procedure used to induce this condition in laboratory animals.

It is also known that the condition called breast dysplasia is stimulated by taking the hormone. And, in both rats and human beings, Dr. Eskin has shown how iodine deficiency figures in this pathological picture.

Breast dysplasia (abnormal changes in the tissue, nodules, benign tumors, cysts) is not malignant. Most women with this condition—some 25 percent of the adult female population—never get cancer. Yet, in a sense, it could be called precancerous. For, as Dr. Eskin notes, "it is generally accepted that carcinoma occurs 4 times as often in dysplastic breasts as it does in normal breasts." In other words, dysplasia *can* develop into cancerous growth.

And through his animal experiments, Dr. Eskin has definitely established that iodine deficiency accompanies dysplasia. Furthermore, the effect of the deficiency on breast dysplasia is greatly augmented by administering estrogen at the same time. The combination of the two causes far more damage than either one by itself.

Definitely encouraging, on the other hand, is the fact that the dysplasia yields to iodine therapy. The condition gradually improves and reverses when the animal is given a high-iodine diet. Iodine is active in the breast tissue itself, as you might surmise. Through quantitative measurement, Dr. Eskin has shown that the amount of iodine in the breast is inversely related to the extent of dysplasia. Rats that measured lowest in breast-iodine content were those that showed dysplasia in the severest form.

Thus far, in Dr. Eskin's work with human subjects, the lessons of the laboratory seem to apply. He writes of ten dysplasia cases— five of whom had their first discomfort after starting on estrogen. All ten women were tested objectively for breast lesions with both mammography (x-ray) and thermography (an extremely sensitive measure of heat, an indication of tissue growth). Thyroid activity was also tested as an indication of iodine status.

After adequate iodine therapy, Dr. Eskin recounts, the tests were given again. In all cases the condition had decreased or disappeared. "The treatment," he states, "seemed to be effective and at least temporarily improved the breast condition. There is need for further basic information on these therapeutic regimes and longer periods of follow-up on these patients."

In light of his studies, Dr. Eskin has become convinced that iodine inadequacy is a cause in progressive breast disease and induced carcinoma. Sex hormones have a profound effect on the mammary gland, he says.

And the best way to protect your breasts against residues of sex hormones in the meat you eat is to make certain you are not deficient in iodine.

The easiest way to do that is to use iodized salt if you are able to consume a fair amount of salt without its harming you. If you have high blood pressure or if your tissues accumulate water in the week before menstruation, you may be better off cutting down on your salt intake, which is a good way to rid your body of surplus water. If you have these or other reasons for avoiding salt, then you ought to know about kelp.

Kelp is a seaweed that is dried and powdered and sold to the consumer as a food flavoring. You can use it as a salt substitute. It does have some salt in it, but much less than the equivalent amount of table salt. It is rich in iodine as well as other sea-water minerals, and its flavor is pleasant.

I might add that in Japan, where the rate of breast cancer is so sensationally low, seaweed is a staple of the diet.

In the Borden Company's *Review of Nutrition Research* (1966) it is pointed out that to get 100 micrograms of iodine (estimated as the normal daily requirement for human beings) one would have to eat

10 pounds of fresh vegetables and fruits, or
 8 pounds of cereals, grains and nuts, or
 6 pounds of meat, fresh-water fish, fowl, or
 2 pounds of eggs, or
 .3 pounds of marine fish, or
 .2 pounds of shellfish.

The review goes on to state: "The problem of obtaining sufficient iodine from food of non-marine origin may be seen from values shown in this table. Iodine-rich seaweed is an abundant source on a limited scale for some peoples. Kelp contains about 200,000 micrograms per kilogram and the dried kelp meal nearly ten times as much, or .1 per cent to .2 per cent of iodine. Used as a condiment this would provide ten times as much iodine as American iodized salt."

The DES residues in meat are much smaller than the quantities of estrogen taken by women who use oral contraceptives, yet there is a distinct possibility that they are contributing and will contribute much more in the future to the alarmingly increasing rate of breast cancer particularly. At present some 74,000 women a year have been developing this form of cancer, and 33,000 are dying of it. The rate has been increasing and may be expected to go on increasing.

Nor is there much reason to doubt the role of DES. David Hawkins, a researcher for the Natural Resources Defense Council, which has filed suit to stop the use of this hormone, said that seventeen men who took DES as a treatment for prostate cancer subsequently developed breast cancer, a disease rare in males (Washington *Post,* October 24, 1971).

Warnings against the use of this potent carcinogen in foods have been made repeatedly, at the Delaney committee hearings on hazardous substances in food before Congress back in the 1950s, by annual meetings of the International Union Against Cancer in 1956, 1962 and 1970 and by scientists and doctors who maintain that even more dangerous than an occasional large dose of stilbestrol, such as was taken by the women whose daughters suffered vaginal cancer, is the hazard of repeated small amounts—in other words, what you get with your daily meat.

The statistics seem to keep getting worse, but you don't have to be one of the numbers in the wrong column. Just see that there is always enough iodine in your diet.

And the best source for iodine in your diet is kelp. Unlike fish, which are also rich in iodine, seaweed is at the bottom of the food chain and does not accumulate pollutants as do the higher forms of life. You can get kelp in tablets or powder—a very small addition indeed to your daily supplements, but one that just might pay off in tremendous dividends. Many people use it regularly as a salt substitute and find the flavor delightful; incidentally they have been providing themselves with the spectrum of trace minerals, never in quantities great enough to have a toxic effect, and consuming sufficient iodine to protect their breasts.

18 Just a Little Cancer

The Delaney amendment to the Food, Drug and Cosmetics Law is either famous or notorious, depending on your point of view. It provides for banning from the food supply any substance shown to cause cancer in test animals. Ordinary consumers can bless the name of James J. Delaney for making it a little bit safer to eat our food. Those who produce additives such as cyclamates, though, feel differently about the Congressman from New York and his amendment. They are now pushing a concerted drive to weaken or eliminate the amendment.

How does Delaney himself feel about his anti-cancer amendment, fifteen years after its passage?

Not only should our food law be maintained, says Delaney—it must be strengthened and fully enforced. "Sure, I think there will be more stopped than cyclamates and DDT," he remarked in a personal interview. "If there's extensive investigation, many things now regarded as safe will be found dangerous."

It could hardly be otherwise. There are some twenty-five hundred chemical substances routinely being added to our daily food, in the estimate of G. O. Kermode writing in the March, 1972, issue of *Scientific American*. They are being used as flavorings, colorings, preservatives, emulsifiers, stabilizers and anything else you can think of that can be done to a food to make it cheaper to manufacture, easier to sell and longer-lived on the market shelf. They are added in microscopic quantities, but they do accumulate.

It is generally agreed that from our normal diets we each eat five pounds of chemicals a year. And, as the Food, Drug and Cosmetic Act is written and interpreted, these chemicals get the same judicial benefit as a man on trial—they are presumed innocent until people start dropping from their consumption.

Food processors are compelled to feed their additives to test animals and report any incidence of cancer, which is sufficient grounds for banning the additive under the provisions of the Delaney amendment. Cancer is a tricky as well as a deadly disease, however. We have seen in discussing DES that large doses of the carcinogen administered by doctors only showed up as cancer in the daughters of their patients twenty years later. In test animals the disease may make no appearance in the three generations tested, only to occur in the fifth or sixth generation, after testing has ceased. And many of the hundreds of thousands of new cancer cases every year may well have been caused by chemicals that were eaten in food twenty or thirty years ago—but there is no way on this earth to prove it.

Thus it is perfectly possible for tests to "prove" that an additive like sodium cyclamate (remember that sudden banning of diet drinks?) does not cause cancer, and then, after the chemical has been in common use for fifteen years, have fresh evidence suddenly turn up establishing that it can cause cancer and may have been doing so all along.

Actually, our food supply is loaded with chemicals that may well be carcinogenic, though the case against them has not yet been made. The best thing to do is avoid them whenever possible. In some cases, however, it is also possible to provide yourself with some protection.

You will recall our discussion of how nitrates get into our drinking water from fertilizer runoff and how they are transformed into cancer-causing nitrites. The same pollutants are deliberately added to food.

Both nitrate and nitrite compounds are heavily used as food preservatives, particularly in smoked fish and processed meats, such as hot dogs, luncheon meats, cured ham and corned beef. Most shockingly, their preservative quality is not particularly necessary today since other compounds have been developed that can do the job as well or better. But the food industry, with the sanction of the Food and Drug Administration, clings to the nitrous preservatives on the claim that they are necessary to prevent botulism. There is a smattering of truth in this claim, but the chemicals are added to food in quantities that have nothing to do with preventing botulism and everything to do with giving the meats their salable red color. People will buy more red hot dogs than gray or brown ones. On such arbitrary preferences our modern plagues may hinge.

All in all, through its hopped-up use of nitrates and nitrites, our society has devised the perfect way to skyrocket the incidence of cancer, even if the proof is not yet so definitive as to compel the FDA to ban the additives.

A group of scientists at the University of Nebraska and Harvard state that nitrosamines are manufactured in the stomach through the combination of dietary nitrite and any of a number of secondary amines. In other words, we can and do synthesize our own carcinogens if our diet includes an unlucky combination of these two substances. This information was presented in an article in *Nature* (January 3, 1970) by Dr. William Lijinsky, of the University of Nebraska's Eppley Institute for Research in Cancer, and Dr. Samuel Epstein, environmental pathologist and toxicologist at Harvard.

In their quest to find an environmental factor that could lie behind the high incidence of cancer, Dr. Lijinsky and Dr. Epstein sought "the perfect carcinogen"—that is, a compound that is widespread and induces tumors in many different organs in many animal models. The nitrosamines, first discovered as carcinogenic in 1956, seemed to fill the bill in most respects. For example, one of the nitrosamines (dimethylnitrosamine) causes tumors in the livers, stomachs, esophagi and noses of mice and in the livers of guinea pigs, rabbits, dogs, monkeys, fish and hamsters. Another (nitrosomethylurea) causes tumors of the liver, skin, brain, spinal cord, lungs, intestines, adrenals, bladder, kidneys and several other organs.

Speaking to the Environmental Mutagen Society in Washington on April 4, 1970, Dr. Lijinsky said: "The findings so far show that nitroso compounds [nitrosamines] are able to elicit tumors in almost all organs and tissues. There is no reason to suspect that man is immune to their action."

As for the presence of secondary amines in the environment, Dr. Lijinsky and Dr. Epstein say the information about their distribution is scant. They speculate that the cooking of meats and fish might release certain free amino acids which, in a series of chemical reactions, could, in the presence of nitrite in the stomach, result in carcinogenic nitrosamines.

They also point out that secondary amines are found in tobacco and fish meal and are used by the food industry for a number of purposes, including flavoring. Of the three amines used by the Nebraska researchers in the experiment that produced cancer tumors in mice, one (morpholine) is a permitted food additive in trace quantities for canned food cooked with steam; it is added to the water in boilers to protect the metal against corrosion. It is also permitted as an anti-fungus spray on fruits and vegetables.

The two scientists logically recommend a "reduction in human exposure to nitrites and certain secondary amines, particularly in foods"—a reduction which they say "may result in a decrease in the incidence of human cancer." Quite simply, the two believe that in nitrosamines we may have found the underlying cause of many human cancers. "On the immediate practical level," they suggest, "it should not be difficult to reduce the amount of nitrite and nitrate added as preservatives to food, particularly meat and fish."

But in this suggestion the researchers make what is probably their only inaccurate statement. Not *difficult* to eliminate a food additive to which the industry is devoted? Not *difficult* to make the FDA see the light and ban (or even lessen) the use of nitrites and nitrates?

For in answer to the dangers outlined by Dr. Lijinsky and Dr. Epstein, FDA's associate director for science, Dr. Dale Lindsay, said: "We don't need the nitrites [as a preservative] nearly as much as we once did. But color is now an important part of a processed meat product. . . . The nitrites are safe at the indicated maximum levels until proved otherwise." When evidence was again presented on the production of tumors in mice fed amines and nitrite, FDA commissioner Charles Edwards told a press conference on November 14, 1971, that "nitrosamines present no imminent hazard and no reduction is required in the amount of nitrite allowed in food."

It seems pretty obvious that the nitrates and nitrites are going to stay in foods until the medical profession turns up authenticated cases of people who developed cancer as a result of eating hot dogs or smoked whitefish, and those cases are established beyond dispute. I'd suggest that you try not to be one of them.

The best thing to do, of course, is curb your appetite for preserved meats. If you never eat smoked fish, hot dogs, salami or other sausages or canned meats you can stop worrying about this hazard. If you can't resist them or must eat them, take some vitamin C every time you do. This, you may recall, is the recommendation of some of the country's top cancer specialists.

The nitrates, which merely cause high blood pressure, and their lethal cousins the nitrites are, however, only a tiny fraction in the five pounds of food chemicals we each consume yearly. Equally deadly in potential are a number of color additives which serve no purpose except to tint foods one or another shade of red, the color that technicians have found will give a food the greatest sales appeal.

One such chemical is a government "certified," or approved, food, drug and cosmetic (FD&C) colorant called Red No. 2. Its real name is amaranth, and it is a sodium salt which contains sulfur and naphtha. Last year a million and a half pounds of it were dumped into foods that cost consumers $10 billion, making it the most commonly used artificial food and cosmetic colorant. It is the chemical to which Dr. Sidney M. Wolfe of Ralph Nader's Health Research Group referred when he told Food and Drug Administration Commissioner Charles Edwards in 1972, "Further inaction or action short of complete removal of FD&C Red No. 2 is inexcusable and should incur legal sanctions to those responsible."

It's not that the FDA isn't aware of the danger. As reported by Victor Cohen in the February 11, 1972, Washington *Post,* Dr. Virgil O. Wodicka, head of the FDA's bureau of foods, "forecast 'some limits' soon on Red No. 2 but 'probably' not a complete ban unless tests still under way show the situation to be more alarming than FDA believes." The FDA is pretty tough to alarm.

How did this health hazard get on the market to begin with? The Washington *Post* on November 14, 1971, briefly explained, "The FDA 'provisionally' listed it in 1960 and was to have made a final determination of safety by December, 1962, but never had done so." In other words, the FDA certified the dye before it was proven safe, and then actually neglected its own follow-up investigation entirely.

The food industry is certainly convinced that profits depend on giving food a bright, unnatural red color. For years Red No. 2 has been liberally used to color lipstick, toothpaste, mouthwash, sodas, fruit drinks, candy, confections, pet foods, bakery goods, ice cream, sherbet, sausage, jams and jellies, gelatin, cereals, dairy products and maraschino cherries.

So if our government food-protection agency seemed satisfied with this coal-tar dye, who sounded the alarm? The name notwithstanding, it was Russian scientists who fingered Red No. 2.

The Russians subjected the colorant to varied and rigorous testing and came up with several different, and all unfavorable, discoveries about what American children have for years been charmed by in their breakfast cereals, their sodas, and their strawberry ice cream and gelatin desserts.

They noted birth defects among animals after pregnant females were fed the colorant, and also reduced litter size as a result of diminished fertility. Later the FDA, according to the October 11, 1971, *Wall Street Journal,* confirmed the findings.

The Soviet scientists also performed a four-year study, published in 1970, in which one group of test animals ate food containing Red No. 2, and another group was given food that did not contain the chemical. Thirteen of the forty-eight rats that ate foods containing the colorant developed tumors, while fifty control animals that did not eat the dye showed no incidence of tumors.

Late in 1971 Ralph Nader and two physicians asked the FDA to halt the use of Red No. 2 immediately on the basis of these studies. And in March, 1972, scientists were still pleading with the FDA to ban that chemical, and several other "certified" dyes as well. Red No. 2 is still in use. It has not been definitively proven to cause cancer and the law does not require the banning of food additives because they induce birth defects. On October 15, 1973, Dr. Albert Kolbye, Jr., deputy director of the FDA Bureau of Foods, told the Agricultural Research Institute in Washington that the FDA is not yet ready to require reporting of potential mutagens and teratogens.

The April 1, 1972, issue of *Health Bulletin* reported, "According to Dr. Michael F. Jacobson, Co-Director of the Center for Science in the Public Interest, if processors quit using the color chemicals just in ice cream, breakfast cereals, hot dogs and pet food, the annual consumption of these suspect compounds would be reduced by better than one million pounds a year, or about one-third." Dr. Jacobson asked that the dye called Orange B also be thoroughly tested before allowing it to be used any more in its primary job of coloring frankfurters. The reason is that the dye, in his words, "is closely related to Red 2 and has not been adequately tested."

The Washington microbiologist also lashed out against Violet No. 1, familiar to every shopper as the "ink" used to stamp the government meat-inspection symbols. He told reporters, "The best animal study indicated that the dye causes cancer, but the FDA rejects the results of this study because it is not known for sure that the dye was pure."

The last of the colorings named by Jacobson is called Citrus Red No. 2. It is added, as the name implies, to oranges to give them a uniform color. Often red-skinned potatoes are given a similar coating of colored wax. The stipulation by law is that consumers are to be informed that coloring has been added to these foods. How many times, though, have you seen a "color added" sign in the vicinity of the supermarket bins containing either oranges or red-skinned potatoes? "A harmless coloring called 'Citrus Red No. 2' is permitted to make oranges more attractive," the FDA stated in a "Student Reference Sheet" in 1965. This chemical, which the FDA assured consumers was "harmless" in 1965, was the same coal-tar dye reported by the *British Journal of Cancer* in 1968 to triple the incidence of bladder cancer in laboratory animals.

When it comes to bladder cancer, it is again vitamin C that would seem to afford us the most protection. But only if we take enough of it. How much? According to Dr. Jorgen U. Schlegel of Tulane University Department of Urology, enough so that it keeps spilling over into your urine.

Cancer of the urinary organs is on the increase. The American Cancer Society estimates that there are some thirty-five thousand new cases every year. Not all of them are due to food dyes, of course. A good many derive from cigarette smoking, being caused by tobacco by-products that are filtered into the urinary bladder for excretion. The same disease is also caused by industrial aniline dyes as well as food dyes.

Dr. Schlegel advises "lots of vitamin C" as the best agent to use against this chemically stimulated cancer. He means more than twenty times the amount recommended for the maintenance of good health by the National Research Council's Food and Nutrition Board, which is 75 milligrams and is considered to be the amount which provides tissue levels approaching saturation *under normal conditions.*

The aim, Dr. Schlegel stated in a telephone discussion, is to exceed the body's requirements so that the excess of ascorbic acid (vitamin C) will spill over into the urine. Dr. Schlegel has studied the effect of massive doses of vitamin C for five years and he and Tulane biochemist George E. Pipkin have been able to demonstrate that, in the presence of ascorbic acid, carcinogenic metabolites will not develop in the urine.

Dr. Schlegel and Dr. Pipkin told the American Association of Genito-Urinary Surgeons in May, 1968, that they could gauge the carcinogenic potential of urine by chemiluminescence, the amount of light generated by high-energy electronic excitation. After his subjects took ascorbic acid for several days, chemiluminescence decreased significantly in all of them.

In their practice the doctors have found that after surgical removal of bladder cancers, they can prevent recurrence with vitamin C. Whether the vitamin can also prevent the cancer would be virtually impossible to prove, but on the basis of their chemiluminescence studies they believe that it will. That's good enough for me. When leading urologists, on the basis of such studies as it is possible to make, tell me that fifteen hundred milligrams of vitamin C a day are my best protection against the type of cancer caused by a variety of food dyes, you know I'm popping vitamin C the way Ronald Reagan pops jelly beans. (And speaking of jelly beans, don't let your kids eat the black ones. They're blackened with lamp black, a known carcinogen that the FDA once considered banning, only to change its mind because it didn't want to deprive the kiddies.)

Nor are the color additives in food the end of the problem. Really, they don't even scratch the surface. Artificial sweeteners, which are used in much greater quantities, are an even bigger problem. There is no point in worrying about sodium cyclamate now, since it has been banned, though the people who used it heavily over a period of years have something to worry about. But the demand for noncaloric sweeteners has hardly diminished, and today saccharin is being used instead, although it has already been found that feeding it to rats produces tumors. In all probability saccharin is just as dangerous as its predecessor.

When you get right down to it, there is just no way of telling how many dozens or hundreds of the twenty-five hundred sanctioned food chemicals may be building our fantastic cancer rate, as well as causing other diseases of which we have even less knowledge, since there is no Delaney amendment requiring testing for them.

Perhaps most significant on the legislative scene is a bill introduced by Wisconsin's dedicated Senator Gaylord Nelson. Under it, food additives would be redefined and the Delaney amendment expanded to require comprehensive testing of additives for a wide range of potential health hazards. Senator Nelson would strike out the language of the existing amendment, changing it to state that *no* food additive is safe if it is found to induce chronic biological injury or damage, including cancer, congenital deformities or genetic mutation, or if it is found after test to induce chronic biological injury or damage in any respect in man or animal. That, says Congressman Delaney, is a big step forward, and he'd like to see the bill passed and put to work.

But, while there is progress, such as the Delaney clause enforcement to halt the cyclamates and to stop the use of cancer-causing estrogens to fatten cattle and caponize roosters, a sharp clash is ahead. A fight in Congress over the clause is already brewing. It's been attacked by both the food industry and the AMA. The trouble with the Delaney amendment, as the major chemical and agricultural interests see it, is that modern techniques of scientific measurement permit us to detect minute traces of chemical residue in food. A zero-tolerance scale for DDT, for example, would exclude from the American diet most meat and fish, and many dairy products. "Well, that's good," counters Delaney. "Let's not have 'business at all costs'—not at the cost of the public's health."

Confirmation of the Delaney-Nelson point of view came in January, 1973, when the New York Academy of Sciences held a meeting to explore whether the Delaney amendment should be scrapped. Overwhelmingly, the scientists at the conference expressed their view that such action would be disastrous, and their strong scientific verdict has served to stay, for the time being, the industrial drive to win tolerance for small quantities of cancer-causing substances in foods.

Nevertheless, we go on drowning in a sea of carcinogens, as the situation was described at the NYAS conference. And, regardless of the value of vitamin C against special chemicals, there is no reason to suppose it can protect us against all of them.

Is there anything else we can do?

The best answer is that it isn't all that necessary to eat processed foods. It is hard to eliminate them completely, of course, but we can avoid preserved meats and stick to what is fresh and untreated. If we buy bread from a small local bakery or bake it ourselves, we can avoid most of the additives designed to give it long life on a market shelf. Fresh vegetables—peas, carrots, potatoes or what have you—are far safer than those that come in cans or packages. The same goes for fruits. It's safer to eat eggs for breakfast than processed cereal. And it's safer, in buying packaged foods, to look for those that proclaim they contain no artificial color, flavors or preservatives.

When you buy fresh fruits and vegetables you have to be sure to wash them carefully to remove any residues of pesticide sprays. That's trouble, of course, but at least you can get rid of the pesticides. The red coloring added to maraschino cherries and frozen strawberries can't be eliminated in any way.

There's no doubt that fresh, whole foods are more trouble to prepare. It is convenience that has made the market for processed foods so enormous. But remember, if you ever come down with a fatal disease because of the chemicals in convenience foods, you will then learn what trouble really is.

There is one additional measure you can take. There is no hard proof of its value, but plenty of suggestive evidence. It is to eat plenty of liver, or else get liver in your diet daily in desiccated-liver supplements.

It has been known since 1951 that desiccated liver, taken every day in sufficient quantity, contains some factor that will prevent cancer that would otherwise be caused by certain chemical carcinogens. Less well known, but even better established scientifically, the same whole-liver product has been found to help the body detoxify a wide variety of chemicals that are indisputably dangerous but extremely hard to escape from.

With a regular intake of enough desiccated liver, the body can detoxify cortisone and thyroid hormone, eliminating frightening side effects, and it has been found to detoxify petroleum hydrocarbons, many pharmaceutical drugs, nicotine, alcohol and marijuana.

Yet, until 1971, all the scientists working with the detoxifying ability of liver had to admit that they just didn't understand what it is about liver that enables it to play this special role. It was not the B-complex vitamins or the minerals with which liver is richly endowed, since, as important as these nutrients are, in themselves they were never found to be able to duplicate the potent protective quality of whole liver. In 1971 in the Department of Biochemistry of the University of Michigan Medical Center, a team of five biochemists headed by the department chairman, Professor Minor J. Coon, succeeded in isolating and subsequently testing a red protein pigment which has been tagged "Cytochrome P-450." And this pigment, extracted from liver, proved itself able to perform all the mysterious protective functions of liver that had been previously found not attributable to the vitamins and minerals liver contains. The important development was reported to the July, 1971, meeting of the British Biochemical Society in Scotland. "P-450 should have been called Miraculase," comments one of Dr. Coon's students.

Small wonder! For this discovery indicates that for all of us, struggling in a sea of health-destroying environmental pollutants, drugs and chemical additives to our food and drink, liver just might be the life preserver for which we have all been searching.

"Cytochrome P-450 may prove to be part of the solution to pollution, drug addiction, alcoholism and even cancer," stated Dr. Coon in a University of Michigan press release dated July 13, 1971.

Twenty years earlier, a series of remarkable experiments took place over several years at the Sloan-Kettering Institute for Cancer Research in New York City. They were described in detail in the *Journal of Nutrition* (July 10, 1951) by Dr. Kanematsu Sugiura, who had a major part in the research. The experiments found that an artificial food-coloring substance, a dye known as "butter yellow," could produce liver cancer in rats within five months. (This poisonous chemical is no longer permitted to be used in the food industry.)

To test the effect of desiccated liver in a cancer-encouraging diet, three groups of rats were put on a diet of rice and butter yellow. In addition, one group was given 10 percent desiccated liver and a second group 2 percent, while a control group of 50 animals was fed only rice and butter yellow. This test successfully demonstrated that desiccated liver prevents liver cancer. All 50 animals in the control group receiving no liver had cancerous livers within 150 days. All of the rats receiving liver had smooth and practically normal livers. But it was found that the 10 percent ration of liver was necessary to offset the disease. Thirty percent of those who received 2 percent had completely healthy livers, but 70 percent had livers with numerous cancer nodules.

In another experiment it was found that whole beef liver was not as effective as dried beef liver in holding down the cancer. This would seem to indicate that the concentrated desiccated liver is better than whole liver for this purpose.

Although the experiments described were done with rats, Dr. Sugiura says in the *Journal of Nutrition* article, "These dietary influences may prove to play a very large part in the causation, prevention and treatment of human cancer."

If this cancer study was not widely followed up—it was not—at least part of the reason for this neglect was that the experimenters themselves had no idea what it was in liver that has this potent cancer-preventing effect. Was it some factor building the body's resistance mechanisms? Was it something like an antitumor drug? How did it work? And what could it be? No one had a clue.

It is only with the isolation and testing of P-450 that we can guess that this red protein which is located in the liver membranes actually is responsible for biochemical changes rendering harmless the chemicals that otherwise would cause cancer, and that is how desiccated liver works to build the body's resistance to cancer.

It is not the only possibility, however. For Nobel laureate biochemist Albert Szent-Györgyi, working independently, has isolated another substance from liver that he believes valuable against cancer. On May 8, 1972, he told his audience at the dedication of the Gordon H. Scott Hall for Basic Medical Sciences at Wayne State University in Detroit that experiments have definitely shown that "the growth of inoculated cancer in mice is strongly inhibited by extracts of liver."

Dr. Szent-Györgyi, who is director of the Institute for Muscle Research at the Marine Biological Laboratory, Woods Hole, Massachusetts, won the Nobel Prize for both medicine and physiology in 1937 for his discovery of the oxidative processes of the cell among other accomplishments. His recent work has focused on isolating from liver extract the anti-cancer substance for which he and his associate Dr. Laszlo G. Egyud have demonstrated the biological activity and which they have dubbed "retine." It is a substance or compound characterized by its ability to retard neoplastic cell division and growth.

Dr. Egyud, formerly of the Lister Institute of Preventive Medicine in London, has shown that the active moiety of "retine" is a compound belonging to the group of chemicals known as alpha-keto-aldehydes. This keto-aldehyde, however, is a latent form, protected against metabolic decomposition by enzymes. A number of synthetic derivatives of the keto-aldehydes were prepared by Dr. Egyud which are also potent anti-neoplastic agents, but their activities are less than that of the natural inhibitor. So effective has this liver derivative proven in the laboratory that Dr. Szent-Györgyi was moved to predict, "We are on the verge of finding the key to curing cancer."

Perhaps. And perhaps not. But, faced with the well-accepted estimate that some 70 percent of all cancer is caused by chemical pollutants in our environment, and knowing we can't escape them all, we have good reason to grasp at any straw we can find. Liver may turn out to be a very strong straw indeed.

19 Home Is No Refuge

Billions of words have made us all aware of what has happened to the air over downtown Los Angeles, the waters of Lake Erie and the food on the supermarket shelves. Rarely, however, do we stop to think how many of the pollution hazards we face are right in our own homes, often created by our own ignorance.

In one rather famous case, an entire family named Benton was laid low during dinner. Mrs. Benton had scrubbed the kitchen floor with a mixture of a bleaching solution and vinegar, a procedure by which she unwittingly manufactured the same lethal chlorine gas that was used during World War I.

When the family recovered—fortunately they did—Mrs. Benton had thoroughly learned the first principle of trying to keep the air of your home livable: never mix household chemicals unless you know exactly what you are doing and what the result will be.

Although this is one of the more dramatic cases illustrating the effects of indoor air pollution, all our homes are polluted by gases and poisons to some degree. Dr. Igho H. Kornblueh, head of the department of physical medicine and rehabilitation at the University of Pennsylvania, believes that indoor air pollution is a serious problem. Dr. Kornblueh, who has studied this subject for more than twenty years, says, "The air inside an average home is actually more polluted than the air outside it."

The indoor atmosphere is loaded with junk, no doubt about that. Cleaners, bleaches, heated cooking fat and oil and aerosols of all kinds emit vapors that may or may not be harmful. Deaths when youngsters inhaled aerosol sprays "for kicks" have been well publicized, but what happens to all of us when we breath imperceptible amounts of deodorants, disinfectants, cleaners, polishes and other liquids and aerosols used inside the home?

Although industry scientists are quick to point out that some components of sprays can kill if inhaled directly, they contend that smaller amounts dispersed throughout an entire house probably won't injure normal persons. Dr. Kornblueh disagrees vehemently. "No one knows what effect aerosols have when they are mixed together or even sprayed individually," he observes. In fact, the written warning on the sides of many sprays indicate they are dangerous to some parts of the anatomy during normal use. And, although the human respiratory system does have a marvelous capacity for cleansing itself, repeated assaults can weaken it and make it easy prey for pollution-aggravated diseases.

Despite their suspicions, medical authorities have no direct proof of a cause-and-effect relationship between indoor air pollution and disease. The reason: there have been no comprehensive, coordinated, well-funded studies of the problem, although many of the 300,000 toxic or potentially toxic trade-name consumer products are of the types that contribute to indoor air pollution. Miffed by the lack of study, Kornblueh complains, "The government and everyone else pay attention to pollution of the outdoors but not to pollution inside homes and other buildings."

Joining the Penn researcher in calling for an investigation of indoor air pollution is D. M. Vincent Manson, acting chairman of the department of mineralogy at the American Museum of Natural History. Manson contends in *Science Digest* (November, 1972) that pollution in the home should be studied because it is "the microsized example of the outside environment. Problems that exist in modern cities exist in a smaller scale in the home."

The Home Ventilating Institute, which is also concerned about indoor air pollution, claims that indoor air pollution is even *worse* than the outdoor variety. That is because pollutants cannot disperse in a home the way they do out-of-doors. For example, each year industry, homes and motor vehicles pour more than 142 million tons of garbage into the atmosphere, but they disperse relatively quickly—barring freak weather conditions such as the 1966 East Coast temperature inversion. On the other hand, the relatively stagnant air in a home prevents pollutants from escaping.

The Ventilating Institute estimates that if all the grease-laden moisture given off in an average kitchen in the course of a year were collected and bottled each family would end up with nearly twenty-five gallons of residue at year's end. If you don't believe it, just take a quick look at your exhaust fan. According to Dr. Kornblueh, "These substances mixed with emanations from gas stoves are only slightly irritating." However, he questions the long-term effects of such irritation.

Other researchers are going beyond Kornblueh's conclusions. Dr. Theron G. Randolph, an allergist at Henrotin Hospital in Chicago, who is also a pioneer in an evolving branch of allergic medicine known as clinical ecology, claims that indoor air pollution can be far more hazardous than the outdoor variety, and a Philadelphia research team says that at least one pollutant might cause cancer.

Dr. David A. Cooper, Dr. A. Reynolds Crane and Katherine Boucot reported in the March, 1968, *Archives of Environmental Health* that some lung cancer in women might be the result of inhaling vaporized cooking fat and oil. In a study involving nearly fourteen hundred lung-cancer patients, they found that only 1 percent of the males were nonsmokers. However, 41 percent of the women patients were nonsmokers. Obviously, cigarettes couldn't be blamed for every case of lung cancer; moreover, another study showed that cooks have a high incidence of cancer of the respiratory tract. Dr. Cooper, Dr. Crane and Miss Boucot concluded by strongly implicating cooking fats and oils as a carcinogen. They said, "Women are probably not exposed as much as men to air pollutants nor to industrial carcinogens, but are exposed to heated fats and oils in cooking."

Unfortunately, such statistical evidence, no matter how convincing, does not carry much weight with pathologists. Dr. Marvin Kuschner, professor of pathology at New York University, says, "I cannot look at diseased lung tissue and say, 'This is 50 percent air pollution.' Records may tell me that this person lived in the city and smoked cigarettes, but I cannot see it. The changes are not identifiable as originating from a particular cause. The pathologist requires specific markers (chemical particles, disease organisms) to attribute morbid conditions to particular causes. In cases where these markers are absent, one is dependent upon the kind of meticulous epidemiological studies which, for example, established the causal relationship between cigarette smoking and lung cancer."

Nevertheless, the absence of meticulous epidemiological studies of a cause-effect relationship does not rule out cooking fats as a possible cause of lung cancer in women. The fact that 41 percent of the women patients were nonsmokers is significant, and scientists do know that many types of lung disease including cancer can be caused by the oxidation of lipids in the lungs. It is reasonable to assume, then, that daily exposure to vaporized fat or oil might well produce or contribute to disease. And it makes sense to protect yourself by doing less frying in the first place, by always running the exhaust fan when you do fry, and even by wearing a gauze mask over your face when you have to be near cooking fat or oil. You can get them at the drugstore. They are cheap enough to be thrown away after use.

Dr. Randolph, who believes gas appliances are the worst polluters in the home, says that dirty household air can produce effects ranging from mild insomnia, slight anxiety and fatigue to manic behavior, amnesia and schizophrenia. Dr. Randolph's solution is strikingly simple; if they affect you, get rid of the offending gas appliances.

According to Randolph, people can react to natural gas the same way allergy victims react to ragweed, orange juice or certain other foods. Over the past fifteen years, the Henrotin allergist has ordered gas appliances removed from the homes of two thousand highly susceptible victims. Dr. Randolph also emphasizes that emissions from gas appliances are not the only sources of indoor air pollution. Common pesticides, paints, sponge-rubber bedding and furniture and plastics also befoul the air we breathe.

How these pollutants can combine to make life miserable was explained by Dr. Randolph to a medical meeting in London. The case involved a middle-aged woman with a history of fatigue, headaches, constipation, muscle and joint aches, chest pains, numbness in the extremities, profuse perspiration, irritability and depression. Said Dr. Randolph, "There was some improvement after the elimination of the gas kitchen range, the avoidance of specifically incriminated foods, and chemical additives and contaminants of food, but she again worsened after the coal-burning warm-air furnace was converted to gas combustion.

"Improvement occurred after moving to a new home constructed and furnished with the aim of controlling domiciliary air pollution. However, severe headache and depression and related symptoms recurred immediately after a tenant in the basement apartment used an insecticide bomb. Despite much cleaning, scrubbing, and repainting, several months were required before the clinical effects attributed to the insecticide subsided."

Here are some other common contaminants of the household environment that few have ever identified with pollution, but which meet all these criteria: they are put there by man, they are unnatural and they endanger health.

One in every five color television sets in use in the United States is emitting x-rays at a level that has been proven harmful to human beings. And *all* color television sets give off at least some of the rays.

Those figures are a conservative extension of findings of a survey of five thousand Long Island homes with color televisions. The study was conducted by the Suffolk County Public Health Service in cooperation with the United States Public Health Service.

Color TV sets from thirty-seven leading manufacturers were examined, and at least one of each brand was found to be giving off radiation at levels in excess of the danger point set by the National Council on Radiation Protection and Measurement in 1960.

Robert DeVore, an official with the United States Public Health Service's Bureau of Radiological Health, was quoted in the *New York Times* (April 8, 1969) as saying that the Suffolk County Survey is the most far-reaching yet conducted in the United States. As a result, it established radiation danger posed by color TVs as being considerably more serious than previously thought. In the past, it had been estimated that about 225,000 homes in the United States had too much TV radiation. The Suffolk study indicates that the figure should be about 3,000,000.

Concern about the dangers posed by TV radiation gained momentum in 1967 when the General Electric Company recalled more than 100,000 sets because they produced excess radiation. Prior to that, John Nash Ott, an expert on light radiation in environmental health, succeeded in prompting Florida Congressman Paul Rogers to call for a congressional hearing on the potential danger to television viewers from the radiation from color sets. After studying the problems carefully, Ott told a presidential committee that it was vital "to insure that nobody, and especially an infant, remain within 15 feet of any part of an operating television set even if it is in another room." X-radiation easily penetrates most materials, and Ott was especially concerned for children sleeping in beds on the other side of the wall from the television set.

"The infant would receive the full effect of radiation from the least protected part of the set at a stage in its life when radiation could do irreparable damage," he said.

Even before they're born, children can be affected by radiation. Dr. Karl Z. Morgan, director of the Health and Physics Division in Oak Ridge National Laboratory, told a House subcommittee in October, 1967, that the number of childhood deaths from leukemia and other cancers is about 40 percent higher among children whose mothers received diagnostic x-rays during pregnancy. Can color TV have the same effect?

Yes, according to Ott. For example, the recalled General Electric sets were giving off eight roentgens per hour. That is as much radiation as you would get in eight different x-ray exposures!

Senator E. L. Bartlett of Alaska, according to the August 13, 1966, *Health Bulletin,* said that scientists estimate that a person loses two and one-half days of life for every roentgen of x-radiation he receives. If that statement is even nearly correct, it is easy to understand why there is such concern about television sets that emit up to eight roentgens per hour—on already ill hospital patients, as well as those sick at home, and the rest of us, for that matter.

Another common result of excess radiation, especially to the gonads, is genetic damage. When the pattern of the genes is upset, the frequent result is the birth of a dead or grossly deformed child. When your dentist x-rays your jaw, he carefully shields your lap with a lead apron. What shields your sex organs and glands when you watch color TV?

Though this may come as a shock, especially to youngsters, television is not necessary to survival. All TVs give off some radiation, even black-and-white ones. The smart parent will limit TV viewing to an hour or two a day—and it will definitely not be a color TV. Also, the children will be required to sit higher than the screen—the x-ray waves are usually emitted toward the floor—and at least ten feet from the set.

With such simple precautions, which also have their value in preserving sanity, x-ray exposure from TV can be minimized and in all probability will have no consequences other than the usual effects on your nervous system.

"The noise is driving me crazy." This oft-heard remark is not always an idle complaint. It can happen. It is happening with more frequency every year as our homes become increasingly mechanized. And not only can noise pollution cause frazzled nerves, it can affect your hearing, your heart, your digestion and your love life.

Sources of noise pollution are operating right in your own home, where many household devices operate at surprisingly high levels of sound intensity. The effects may well be deleterious to health, says Dr. Lee E. Farr, in an article in the *Journal of the American Medical Association* (October 23, 1967), in which he makes a point of calling the attention of physicians to the role played by noise in provoking disease.

While much attention has been given to the effects of noise in industry during the past thirty years, and maximum levels of industrial sound intensity have been carefully defined, little attention has been paid to the effects of noise in the home. And if, as a member of the affluent society, you have decreased your work with a dishwasher, garbage disposal, washing machine, dryer, ventilating fan, air conditioner, stove vent fan, vacuum cleaner, mixing machine and electric razor, then your home is jumping with noise. Have you perhaps noticed more emotional upsets lately? Noises have been associated with an increase in tension diseases. In fact, says Dr. Farr, noise is so upsetting emotionally that it frequently leads to outbursts of fury or threats, and leaves frustration in its wake.

Many of us tend to dismiss noise as a petty nuisance, something which, because it is intangible, can do no physical harm. But it isn't so. Noise affects both your psyche and your soma—your mind and your body. In the physical sense, noise or sound is actually a vibration of the air, mechanical radiant energy transmitted by pressure waves. In fact, physicists say that sound is actually a result of this vibration on your inner ear; that should a volcano erupt on an uninhabited island, there would be a giant vibration but no sound unless there was an ear to hear it—to convert the vibration into sound. When intense and constant, these vibrations can cause a host of disturbances not only in hearing acuity but also causing many physiologic ailments—migraine headaches, gastrointestinal disorders, fatigue, and an actual lessening of sexual potency. A leading Japanese researcher has found that noise can upset the body's endocrine function, particularly the pituitary-gonadal system, that it causes a thickening of the basal membrane and has an adverse effect on testicular function (*Mie Medical Journal,* Volume IX, No. 1, 1959). These little-known effects were disclosed by Dr. Hiroshi Sakamota of the University School of Medicine in Tsu, whose extensive research on the effects of noise led him to investigate the health status of the inhabitants of a village located near an airfield for jet planes. More than half the inhabitants of the vicinity of the airfield complained of fatigue, lowered work efficiency, headache, palpitation, stiff shoulder, loss in body weight, sleeplessness and an uncomfortable feeling on getting up. Moreover, says Dr. Sakamota, "in the investigation of their sexual life, the greater part of those answering complained of decrease in frequency of sexual intercourse."

The endocrinological effects of noise were further borne out by the finding that there was a remarkable decrease in the number of eggs laid by the hens in a poultry farm near the airfield. This fact, says the Japanese scientist, confirms the endocrine disturbance. To buttress his findings further, Dr. Sakamota, by staining the anterior lobes of the pituitary glands of the hens, demonstrated that this diminished egg laying was due to a decrease in secretion of the gonad-stimulating hormone.

And not only in the village around the jet-plane airfield but also in other places where noise is intense, investigation discloses that people complain of lowered work efficiency, headache, palpitations and loss of vigor. The fact that noise causes physical changes was noted by a famed ear surgeon, Dr. Samuel Rosen of

Columbia College of Physicians, who observed that an unexpected or unwanted noise causes the pupils to dilate, the skin to pale, the mucous membranes to dry, the intestines to go into spasms, and the adrenals to explode secretions (*Annals of Otology, Rhinology, and Laryngology,* September, 1962).

Acoustical engineers measure sound in units called decibels. A level of fifty decibels is considered in the quiet range, and is about what one would find in a living room where no appliances are operating, and the family is engaged in a pleasant conversation. We can live with much louder sound if it is pleasant, such as music. Unpleasant sound will arouse ill effects which can be emotional, physical or a combination of both.

When the vacuum cleaner is in operation, it produces a noise (defined as unwanted sound) of seventy-three decibels. It is interesting to note that the noises which cause emotional trauma are generated by the acts of another and those over which the captive listener has little control. The woman operating the vacuum cleaner may not mind the noise, but it can be a great source of annoyance to her husband. For example, says Dr. Farr, who is director of nuclear medicine at the University of Texas, a patient who goes to his doctor with a bleeding ulcer may recall that the attack came during an argument with his wife. He may overlook the fact that the noise of the vacuum cleaner upset him so that he was itching for an argument. Or was it the jangle of the disposal and the dishwasher in concert with the ventilating fan that triggered his ugly mood? Of course, the shoe can also be on the other foot and there are times when the noise of *his* power saw vibrating in the basement can drive *her* to distraction.

Some families may find that simply changing their furnishings will provide a noticeable decrease in sound transmission. Wall-to-wall carpeting, upholstered furniture and draperies all help to absorb sounds that would be deflected by smoother surfaces. Wood paneling is an excellent sound absorber. Ceilings covered with acoustical tile will absorb as much as 75 percent of all sound.

If you are fortunate enough to be able to plan for the construction of your own home, make sure that the interior walls are built according to the strictest sound-absorbing specifications. These walls should have double rows of studs, staggered and separated by fibrous glass insulation or a "noise stop board"—a piece of hard wallboard suspended in the open space so that it will vibrate slightly and absorb some of the sound. The same effect is possible in ceilings; a false ceiling leaving a small open space where a piece of gypsum board can be mounted on resilient clips will also provide an extra layer for sound absorption.

The floor plan of the home should provide for staggered interior doorways instead of doorways facing directly across hallways. Doors should be well fitted. A gasket to prevent the door from slamming eliminates one very irritating source of nervous strain.

Sound-absorbing wall materials in the washer-dryer area will cut down on annoyances from these work savers, and setting these machines and any others that vibrate on cushioned pads and having them bolted to the floor will bring the noise level down still more. A garbage-disposal unit will be less noisy if it has flexible rather than rigid hose connections.

Outdoors, hedges and trees shield us somewhat from such environmental disturbances as traffic, sirens and jets.

The considerate housewife who is aware of the deleterious effects of noise can do much to protect her husband. She can do her vacuuming and her laundry when he is not at home. If the noise of the dishwasher is a particular annoyance, she can stack the dinner dishes in the evening, add the breakfast dishes next morning and run the machine after her husband has left for the office. She can also refrain from nagging, another source of noise that is hard to turn off and can be the root cause of many physical ailments, says Dr. Farr. "The home environment is one in which we are not concerned primarily with efficient work conditions," he says, "but with effective rest, renewal of vigor and enthusiasm, and the development of a sense of well-being which lead to the establishment and continuance of warm personal bonds within the family and among friends."

Since noise plays such an important role in the family's well-being, the housewife should look to the sounds in the home as carefully as she does to the family's nutrition. While eliminating those noises that are unwanted or intrusive, she should promote those sounds which create a warm reassuring atmosphere—the sound of music in the background, the sound of a singing bird, the sound of laughter and the sound of pleasant voices.

You can find other hazards in some pretty unexpected places in your home environment.

Under some circumstances, the patient of Dr. Bruce Bower, a Hartford, Connecticut, internist, would have been considered perfectly healthy. She was pretty and had a fully developed figure. Her menstrual cycle was a bit irregular, but that is very common in some women. But one thing was rather surprising. Bower's patient was only three years old!

The maturing process had been rapid and painless for the little girl. In six months she changed from a normal-looking three-year-old to what came very close to resembling an attractive teenager. She had grown taller, more shapely, with sparse pubic hair growth and even a more mature personality.

Bower had his patient admitted to Connecticut's Hartford General Hospital and immediately performed a whole battery of tests. The only unusual finding was that the girl's body contained a high saturation of estrogens—so high, in fact, that it was similar to the level expected in normal adult women.

Further tests showed that the girl's body could not have been producing that level of hormones. She must have been absorbing them from somewhere in the environment. She was released from the hospital, and the arduous task of tracking down the source of the hormones was begun. For months, everything the girl ate or came in contact with was analyzed, but still the source was not found. Day by day, she continued to mature.

Bower and his associates grew desperate in their frustration. Permanent hospitalization was seriously considered. But fortunately one day the girl's mother made what she thought was a casual statement to Dr. Bower.

She told him that once a month she and her daughter visited the child's grandmother. While there, the older woman gave the girl her facial cream to play with. "Of course," she said, "that couldn't have anything to do with *this*." She gestured to her daughter's adult figure.

But immediately Dr. Bower knew he had the answer. The jar of cream was brought to his office. He found that each ounce contained ten thousand units of estrogen. Upon further study, it was learned that the child had eaten one-quarter ounce of the cream over a five-month period.

At the time Bower handled this case, it had been the consensus among physicians that a person could swallow two ounces a month of estrogen cream without any harmful effects. Yet the child had eaten only one-fortieth of that amount—and the symptoms were well developed.

Although the child has not yet returned to normal, two years later when her case was reported she had lost most of the obvious signs of what doctors term "isosexual precocity." She is fortunate. A combination of circumstance and a perceptive physician led to an accurate diagnosis. But there are undoubtedly other cases similar to this which remain undiagnosed.

"Labeling these products as potential health hazards or limiting their dissemination is clearly indicated," Dr. Bower told a June, 1972, American Medical Association meeting in San Francisco. Without question, according to Bower, cosmetics pose a public health hazard. The least a woman can do about them is shut them safely away from children.

The hazard is not limited to face creams containing hormones. In October, 1967, the American Medical Association and the Society of Toxicology co-sponsored a symposium on "The Evaluaation of Safety of Cosmetics" in Washington, D.C. One of the speakers at that meeting, Dr. Paul Lazar of Northwestern University Medical School, showed actual slides of men and women whose arms, backs, faces and legs were terribly disfigured by cosmetic products used every day by most people. If anyone doubted the dangers some cosmetics pose, Lazar made it clear: "If there were no reactions to cosmetics, there would be no reason to have this conference at all!"

Some of the victims had large red blots over the parts of their bodies not covered by clothing. Some of the faces were disfigured almost beyond recognition. Others were covered with large scabs or scales. Almost all the cases were photodermatoses—chemical reactions between particular cosmetics and the ultraviolet rays from the sun. These reactions usually occur only in people who are peculiarly allergic to the combination of chemical and sun.

But who are these people? How rare are they? Science cannot answer those questions. But one thing is quite obvious, at least to the dermatologists at the Washington meeting: the number of people susceptible to photoallergic reactions is definitely on the increase.

Most frequently the reactions are caused by antibacterial detergents and soaps. Dermatologists' offices are sometimes crowded with people who, during the summer, take baths in the morning before sunbathing. In a matter of minutes, the ultraviolet rays of the sun cause the chemicals in the soap to interact with allergens in some people's bodies to cause a minor skin irritation, or in some cases a severe infection, open wound or skin cancer.

Disturbingly, the antibacterial soap fad is, according to one dermatologist at the meeting, producing more than its share of allergic reactions.

So seriously does the Academy of Dermatology consider the antibacterial soaps a hazard that in late 1966 the organization wrote to the FDA urging the agency to require a label on the product to read: "Some people may develop allergic reactions to them . . .

that they have a sensitizing effect on some people . . . and that exposure to the sun may cause eruptions."

Under prompting by the Academy, the FDA quietly prohibited cosmetics makers from using Bithionol in their antibacterial products. The chemical was shown to cause serious photosensitive reactions in a significant number of people. Hexachlorophene was not banned until 1973. And many similar chemicals are still in use. According to Dr. Harry M. Robinson, Jr., a Baltimore dermatologist and chairman of an advisory group of the Academy of Dermatology, "These antibacterial ingredients are entirely unnecessary and our committee found they serve no useful purpose by being included in ordinary soaps."

Another physician, Dr. Silas E. O'Quinn of New Orleans, called on the FDA to "stop the indiscriminate addition of such compounds to so many cleaners, cosmetics and proprietary products."

Although he did not name specific brands, Dr. Stephen Rothman of the Department of Medicine at the University of Chicago has publicly attacked soap makers for their practice of including antibacterial agents in their products. He said at a Society of Cosmetic Chemists meeting in 1967, "Incorporation of pharmacologically active ingredients into cosmetics which are sold across the counter is objectionable because no absorbable drug should be given without control of dosage."

Practically all dermatologists agree that germicidal deodorant soaps are a fake. The germs that are killed will be replenished in two or three hours, and they're not what causes odors in the first place. All you need to get clean is plain soap and water. It's all you should have around your home.

Drugs, which we ordinarily think of as health aids, are one of the commonest of household hazards. It is widely known that drugs—especially aspirin—are responsible for the majority of child poisonings. In 1965, according to the National Clearinghouse for Poison Control Centers of the United States Public Health Service, 3,261 children were poisoned by St. Joseph aspirin, and another 2,402 by Bayer aspirin. Thyroid tablets, Bufferin, birth-control pills and even vitamins are responsible for making drugs the leading poisoner among youngsters.

But these cases would be even more common than they are if it were not for the fact that parents usually do recognize that drugs are poisonous. It is the exception to the rule—though a far too frequent exception—when a bottle of tranquilizers is left on the dresser or when aspirin is found on the kitchen table. Parents know drugs should be put away, and usually it is an oversight rather than a common practice that leaves the drug in a place where a child can find it, eat it, and become another statistic, another death.

Parents are not nearly as concerned over the dangers of common houshold products as they are over drugs. Yet, according to the National Clearinghouse for Poison Control Centers' 1965 study, 1,247 children were poisoned that year by Clorox. Three hundred twenty-five swallowed Old English furniture polish. Ajax was consumed by 269 children, and Top Job by 203. Ammonia, Comet, Pride, Purex and the bug killer Raid were swallowed by over 100 children each. About half these children were hospitalized, and a number died.

Dr. Alan K. Done, professor of pediatrics at the University of Utah, pinpointed a major difference in drug poisonings and poisonings from household products. Addressing the 117th Annual American Medical Association Convention in San Francisco, Done said, "Common household products pose a difficult problem in poisoning: Although involved less commonly than drugs, they are usually accompanied by much less information. Frequently the only information available is the trade name of the product and the purpose for which it was intended."

It is not enough to know that a child has been poisoned or even that he has been poisoned by a laundry detergent. It is frequently not enough even to know the name of the detergent. For one type of poisoning, vomiting ought to be induced immediately. For another, the induction of vomiting could be fatal. Drug labels must carry a list of ingredients, but ordinary household products are not required to do so.

Dr. Done came out strongly in favor of education. He said, in effect, that a mother ought to be taught to see a bottle of poison on her dresser, even though the label says it's fingernail polish. Teach her that the permanent-wave neutralizer on the closet floor might just as well be labeled arsenic, for it is equally deadly. Show her that the colorful can of insecticide under the sink, with its pleasant perfumed odor, can be as effective against her child as it is against the flies and mosquitoes.

Pesticides are, in fact, among the most poisonous household products, and Done discussed them at length. "For most classes of pesticides the range of toxicity is great and relatively high," he said. Inorganic compounds are extremely poisonous—which means that, for a two-year-old, less than a swallow can be fatal. Sometimes, says Done, "these products represent an unnecessary risk, and it is often possible to reduce the hazard to children by substituting products having lesser toxicity and comparable effectiveness." In fact, there is no need to have any pesticides at all in the house. Fly traps and other devices are commonly available to rid the home of flying insects without posing the hazards that are inevitable with pesticides.

When you get right down to it, it's not very hard to be aware of the hazards that modern civilized living has introduced into our homes, and to guard against succumbing to them. With just a little effort you can make your home quieter, more peaceful and safer, a place to rest in and restore yourself so that you can go on battling against the threats of the outside world—and win the battle.

20 A Penny Saved Is a Day of Life

It is seriously to be hoped that reading this book has given no one the impression that it is possible to live with impunity amid growing pollution and escape unscathed. It isn't so. Even though you now know preventives and antidotes for some of the most serious consequences of some of the most dangerous pollutants, there are others for which science is still unable to find any defense. One of them is sulfur dioxide, an acknowledged cause of cancer, that is poured into the air by the burning of low-grade fuel oil. There are hundreds of such chemicals in our air, water and food. Even the consequences of many of them are unknown, not to mention defenses against them.

So, though you may take the measures recommended in this book and will be thus able to retain much better health than would otherwise be your lot, it would be foolish optimism to hope for perfect health or anything approaching it as long as we permit our environment to keep getting dirtier and more chemicalized day by day.

Yet, aside from writing nasty letters to our Congressmen, is there anything we can actually do about it?

Not as much as there should be, I'm afraid. The fact remains, however, that if each of us would at least reduce his own contribution to the overall pollution, it could make a significant dent in the amount of filth contaminating the world as well as the amount getting into our own bodies and damaging them.

How do we do that? Basically, by being frugal—by remembering money and trying to save a little in connection with everything we use, no matter how well we can afford to be wasteful.

I believe frugality is the key, for the simple reason that in every area of pollution, it is what is wasted—what has failed to be used—that makes the problem. It is not consumption in itself—it is not affluence in itself—it is the mistaken belief that we can afford to be wasteful that has created a nightmare world around us. Let me give you some specific examples of what frugality can accomplish, because I think it is urgent that you see just how much power you do have in your own hands and just how much you really can accomplish without lowering the quality of life.

Let's consider, for example, the consumption of electric power. It requires no proof that electric power stations manufacture electricity by burning either soft coal or crude oil, both of which pollute the air with enormous quantities of sulfurous oxides. Experts are beginning to classify the air pollution of cities as being either brown or gray, brown being the color of the air when it is polluted chiefly by automobile exhausts and gray being its color, as in New York and Pittsburgh, when the chief pollutant is sulfur dioxide. So increasing pressure is being put on the electric utilities to burn low-sulfur fuel instead. To this they have a reasonable answer. There just isn't enough low-sulfur coal and fuel oil in the world to make the shift, without reducing the amount of power being produced. But, they say, how can they even think of producing less power when the public keeps demanding more year by year?

Those are weasel words, of course. The same companies that complain about how much power we demand are spending advertising fortunes to persuade us to demand still more. Nevertheless, we remember the power brownouts of past summers when heat waves led to maximum air-conditioner use and there simply was not enough electric power to go around. The only solution the power companies have proposed so far is no solution at all—a wholesale switch to nuclear-fission atomic power plants.

I think we can only say that the solution has not yet been found. And, lacking such a solution, the best thing we can do right now is cut down the demand for electric power. Here are some simple ways that you can use less electric power, enjoy a lower electric bill as a result, and by doing so make some improvement in the quality of our air.

Read more and watch TV less. Turn out the lights when you leave a room. Don't keep floodlights on your house all night unless you're really afraid of burglars. Don't use your washing machine until you have a full load; the same goes for the dishwasher. Dishwashers particularly are easily dispensable. If you want a clean dish to come out you have to practically wash it at the sink before you put it in. Why not just finish the job at the sink and let it go at that? In any case, if you love your dishwasher, accumulate your dishes throughout the day and run it only once.

You can also open cans with a manual can opener and less aggravation than the electric can opener causes. Whether you switch to a Gillette or grow a beard, you can easily do without an electric razor. You can hang your wash in the backyard and give it that wonderful clean smell it gets from drying in the wind and sunlight instead of using your electric dryer.

Can such small economies actually have an effect on the power demand? You bet they can. You'll be amazed at the saving in your electricity bill, and if we could somehow multiply the reduction by sixty million households, the saving would be fantastic. We would even have enough reserve power to run our air conditioners during a heat wave, when we really need them, and thus greatly improve the quality of modern life.

Another way we can work wonders for the quality of the air we breathe is simply to use less paper. I hope you will forgive me for stating the obvious when I point out that paper is made from wood and the wood comes from trees that are cut down. It is the demand for paper far more than any other single factor that is responsible for denuding our forests and thus for the fact that our very oxygen supply is in peril. We need more trees, not fewer, to remove more carbon dioxide from the air and convert it into oxygen, and just about the only practical way that will ever be accomplished is if we all figure out ways to use less paper. How do you do it? You give up paper napkins and return to cloth. You take one newspaper a day instead of two or three. You buy your milk in bottles instead of cardboard containers, and you buy soft drinks without a cardboard carrying case. The point is not to do without paper entirely. That would hardly be possible. But we can all reduce the amount of paper we use and then throw away. We can leave more trees in the world and at the same time cut down on all the smoke engendered by burning all that waste paper in the municipal incinerators.

I might also mention that walking or riding a bike is a great deal cheaper than driving and infinitely better for your health.

When you bought that high-performance car, did you improve or deteriorate the quality of your life? Perhaps you could have done more for yourself and the quality of your life by buying a cheaper car with a smaller engine that runs on cheaper gasoline. You would certainly be $500 to $1,000 richer.

With pure water coming into short supply, you can save a surprising amount of it by putting a brick—yes, brick—into your toilet tank. As simply as that, you will be using nearly a quart less of water every time you flush your toilet. Count how many times you flush it in a day, multiply by 365 and you'll be amazed at how many gallons of water can be saved in a year.

The ways that I have mentioned only scratch the surface, of course. You can easily figure out dozens of others in your own life, using the rule of thumb that if it saves just a little money it is also improving the environment. Buying your beer and soft drinks in returnable deposit bottles instead of disposables, for example, saves only two or three cents a bottle, but it also means less litter, less broken glass, less problem of disposing of bottles, and less bottle manufacture to add its own increment to the dirt. Keeping your house only two degrees cooler in winter will save money on your fuel bills and use less of our dwindling energy reserves, as well as throwing less smoke into the air.

You can go on and on.

What it adds up to is that each of us, without much effort or equipment other than a cheap streak, can make a contribution of some note toward actually reducing the health menaces that surround us.

Enough of us can have a marked effect. But it's going to take time to get enough of us aroused actually to take the necessary steps, just as it's going to take time for all our governments to see what has to be done and do it.

Meanwhile, some are going to die under the onslaughts of universal pollution, and a great many people are going to become chronically ill. It is my earnest hope that the readers of this book will fall into neither category. I am certain that those who take it seriously and protect themselves will remain in the thinning ranks of those in good health.

Suggested Reading

American Chemical Society, Committee on Chemistry and Public Affairs, Subcommittee on Environmental Improvement. 1969. *Cleaning Our Environment, the Chemical Basis for Action.* Washington: American Chemical Society.

Ayres, J. C., ed. 1962. *International Symposium on Food Protection.* Ames: Iowa State Univ. Press.

Cailliet, Greg M. 1971. *Everyman's Guide to Ecological Living.* New York: Macmillan.

Camp, Thomas R. 1963. *Water and Its Impurities.* New York: Reinhold.

Carr, Donald Eaton. 1966. *Death of the Sweet Waters.* New York: Norton.

———. 1965. *The Breath of Life.* New York: Norton.

Farber, Seymour M. 1961. *The Air We Breathe.* Springfield: Thomas.

Gofman, John William, and Tamplin, Arthur M. 1971. *Poisoned Power.* Emmaus: Rodale Press.

Jacobs, Morris B. 1960. *The Chemical Analysis of Air Pollutants.* New York: Interscience.

Jacobson, Michael F. 1972. *Eater's Digest.* Garden City: Doubleday.

Jones, Claire. 1972. *Pollution: The Food We Eat.* Minneapolis: Lerner.

Lee, Douglas H. K., ed. 1972. *Environmental Factors in Respiratory Disease.* New York: Academic Press.

———. 1972. *Metallic Contaminants and Human Health.* New York: Academic Press.

———. 1972. *Multiple Factors in the Causation of Environmentally Induced Disease.* New York: Academic Press.

Lewis, Howard R. 1965. *With Every Breath You Take.* New York: Crown.

Nader, Ralph. 1970. *Vanishing Air.* New York: Grossman.

Pitts, J. N., and Metcalf, R. L., eds. 1969–1971. *Advances in Environmental Sciences.* Vols. 1 and 2. New York: Wiley-Interscience.

Rochester Third International Conference on Environmental Toxicity, 1970. 1972. Springfield: Thomas.

Saltonstall, Richard. 1970. *Your Environment and What You Can Do about It.* New York: Walker.

Schroeder, Henry A. 1971. *Pollution, Profits & Progress.* Brattleboro: Stephen Greene Press.

Stone, Irwin. 1972. *The Healing Factor.* New York: Grosset & Dunlap.

Szent-Györgyi, Albert. 1972. *The Living State.* New York: Academic Press.

Van Tassel, Alfred J. 1970. *Environmental Side Effects of Rising Industrial Output.* Lexington: Heath Lexington Books.

Wellford, Harrison. 1972. *Sowing the Wind.* New York: Grossman.

Williams, Roger J. 1971. *Nutrition Against Disease.* New York: Pitman.

Wilson, Billy Ray. 1968. *Environmental Problems.* Philadelphia: Lippincott.

Wise, William. 1968. *Killer Smog.* Chicago: Rand McNally.

Wolozin, Harold. 1966. *The Economics of Air Pollution.* New York: Norton.

Index

241

Sultz, Harry A., 53, 54
Sunlight, effects of, 64–72
Sussman, Oscar J., 184, 185
Swordfish, 110, 111, 112
Szent-Györgyi, Albert, 28, 30, 97–98, 99, 215, 216; quoted, 99–100

Tappel, A. L., 22–23
Television, x-ray exposure from, 221–222, 223, 224
Thyroid gland, 70, 118, 196
Thyroxine, 118, 196
Tipton, Isabel H., 172
Tomato juice, with desiccated liver, 156
Tooth decay, 70
Tranquilizers, 165, 169, 232
Tuna fish, 110, 111, 112, 114, 115, 116, 170
Typhoid, 73, 74, 75, 78

Ultraviolet rays, 64, 66, 67, 71, 230

Violet No. 1, 209
Vitamin A, 18–19, 32, 35, 59, 60, 98, 119; for asthma, 55, 56, 58; for bronchitis, 15–16, 17, 56; and cilia, 16–17, 55; for dermatitis, 55; infections fought by, 16; as lung cancer preventive, 12–14, 15, 16, 17, 18; and lysosomes, 17–18; mucous membranes maintained by, 15–16, 55; for rhinitis, 55; sources of, 20, 60; toxic reactions to, 19–20; and vitamin E, 32
Vitamin B₁, 118
Vitamin B₃, 135
Vitamin B complex, 118; deficiency of, 118; and heart, 118
Vitamin C, 92, 96, 97, 135, 206; as antioxidant, 93, 99; and bladder cancer, protection from, 209, 210; cadmium detoxified by, 96, 178–180; for colds, 98; deficiency of, 61, 92; detoxifying effects of, 90, 91, 96, 178–179; for hemoglobin formation, 156; and lead damage, protection from, 144–145; and leukocytes, 97; nitrites destroyed by, 89, 90, 97; prickly heat cured

by, 97; recommended in large doses, 93–94, 97, 99; as reducing agent, 90, 99; safety of, 94; and wheat germ, 98, 99, 100
Vitamin C and the Common Cold (Pauling), 92
Vitamin D, 5, 57, 58, 59, 60, 64, 67, 71; for asthma, 55, 56, 58; deficiency of, 60, 61, 62, 63; for dermatitis, 55; for rhinitis, 55; sources of, 62, 63
Vitamin E, 25, 26, 28, 30, 31; as antioxidant, 24, 31, 32; as dietary supplement, 33; fibrin dissolved by, 29; and heart attack, prevention of, 29, 33; and ozone, prevention of effects of, 23–25, 31; Shute's recommendation for, 33; and vitamin A, 32
Voeller, Kytja, 137, 138
Von Oettingen, W. F., 8

Waerland, Ebba, 107
Water: chlorinated, 73–82 *passim;* nitrate in, 83–87 *passim,* 97, 203; pollution of, 73; saving, 237; soft, 175
Weick, Mary Theodora, 61
Weight training, to reduce movement time, 162–163
Wheat germ, 32, 33, 98, 99, 100, 116, 178
White, Paul Dudley, 29, 77, 78
White bread, as worthless food, 170–171
Whole wheat, 189
Williams, Roger J., 19, 170, 171
Wodicka, Virgil O., 207
Wolf, George, 18
Wolfe, Sidney M., 207
Wurtman, Richard, 66, 69, 70

X-rays, 19, 221, 222, 223, 224

Yogurt, 191

Zinc, 171, 175, 176, 177, 178; and cadmium, 172, 173, 174, 175, 180; sources of dietary, 178
Zinc oxide, as pollutant, 9

DATE			